Virtual Medical Office

for

Fordney:
Insurance Handbook for the Medical Office,
12th Edition

Virtual Medical Office

for

Fordney:
Insurance Handbook for the Medical Office,
12th Edition

Study Guide prepared by

Linda Smith, CPC, CPC-I, CEMC, PCS, CAC, CMBS

Healthcare Instructor/Consultant
MedOffice Resources
Greene, New York

Textbook by:

Marilyn Takahashi Fordney, CMA-AC, CMT

Formerly Instructor of Medical Insurance, Medical Terminology,
Medical Machine Transcription, and Medical Office Procedures
Ventura College
Ventura, California

software developed by

Wolfsong Informatics, LLC
Tucson, Arizona

ELSEVIER
SAUNDERS

3251 Riverport Lane
Maryland Heights, Missouri 63043

VIRTUAL MEDICAL OFFICE FOR   ISBN: 978-1-4377-2338-0
FORDNEY:
INSURANCE HANDBOOK FOR THE MEDICAL OFFICE
TWELFTH EDITION
Copyright © 2012, 2010, 2008, 2006, 2004, 2002, 1999, 1997, 1995, 1989, 1981, 1977 by Saunders, an imprint of Elsevier Inc.

Notice

Knowledge and best practice in this field are constantly changing. As new research and experience
broaden our knowledge, changes in practice, treatment and drug therapy may become necessary or
appropriate. Readers are advised to check the most current information provided (i) on procedures
featured or (ii) by the manufacturer of each product to be administered, to verify the recommended
dose or formula, the method and duration of administration, and contraindications. It is the
responsibility of the practitioner, relying on their own experience and knowledge of the patient, to
make diagnoses, to determine dosages and the best treatment for each individual patient, and to
take all appropriate safety precautions. To the fullest extent of the law, neither the Publisher nor
the Authors assumes any liability for any injury and/or damage to persons or property arising out
or related to any use of the material contained in this book.

ISBN: 978-1-4377-2338-0

Acquisitions Editor: Susan Cole
Associate Developmental Editor: Karen Baer
Publishing Services Manager: Pat Joiner-Myers

Printed in the United States of America

Last digit is the print number: 9 8 7 6 5 4 3 2 1

Table of Contents

Reviewers

Jason Belanger, BA, CMAA, CBCS
Instructor
Medical Administrative
Loring Job Corps
Limestone, Maine

Jennifer Flippin, CPC
Medical Billing and Coding Program Coordinator
Medical Billing and Coding
Pinnacle Career Institute
Lawrence, Kansas

Michelle Grant, RHIT
Instructor
Health Information Technology
Northeast Iowa Community College
Peosta, Iowa

Chanda Littleton, CCP, CPC, CBCS, CMAA
Instructor
Healthcare Information Management
New Horizons, Inc.
Durham, North Carolina

Deanne Ulrich, BA, MAE
Instructor
Business and Information Technology/Medical Office
Hawkeye Community College
Waterloo, Iowa

Barbara Wilson, CPC, CCS-P, RHIT
Program Director
Medical Billing and Coding
Southeastern Institute
Charlotte, North Carolina

Getting Started

■ LOGIN AND ENROLLMENT INSTRUCTIONS

Please check with your instructor prior to registering to verify whether you are required to enroll in the instructor's *Virtual Medical Office* course on Evolve. If so, your instructor will provide you with your course ID and you will use the steps under **Instructor-Led Course** on the following page.

SELF-STUDY COURSE

1. To access your *Virtual Medical Office*, go to http://evolve.elsevier.com/Fordney/handbook/.
2. Select the **Simulations—VMO** tab and click **Register for These Simulations** to begin the one-time-only registration process.
3. Select **I already have an Access code** and enter the code located on the inside front cover of this Study Guide exactly as it appears.
4. Click **Register**.
5. If you already have an Evolve account or have previously requested products from Evolve, provide your case-sensitive username and password in the Returning User area and click **Login**. If you do not have an Evolve account, provide your desired password for the account in the New User area and click **Continue**. Provide the required profile information and click **Continue**.
6. Read the Registered User Agreement. Check **Yes, I accept this agreement** and then click **Submit**.
7. A screen confirming your enrollment will appear. Click **My Home**.
8. This product will be added to your Evolve account in the My Content area located on the left-hand side of the Evolve homepage. Click to expand the **Simulations—VMO** heading and then click the link titled **Fordney: Insurance Handbook for the Medical Office, Twelfth Edition**.
9. Click **Simulations—VMO** to access your activities.
10. Your case-sensitive account information will be e-mailed to you. Please note your account information. If needed, you can request your account information at any time by clicking on **I forgot my login information** on the Evolve homepage.
11. Bookmark this page (http://evolve.elsevier.com/student) to easily log in and access your *Virtual Medical Office* in the future.

INSTRUCTOR-LED COURSE

1. Go to http://evolve.elsevier.com/enroll.
2. Enter the **Course ID** provided to you by your instructor and click the arrow button.
3. Verify that the course information is correct and check **Yes, this is my course**.
4. Select **I already have an Access code** and enter the code located on the inside front cover of this Study Guide exactly as it appears.
5. Click **Register**.
6. If you already have an Evolve account or have previously requested products from Evolve, provide your case-sensitive username and password in the Returning User area and click **Login**. If you do not have an Evolve account, provide your desired password for the account in the New User area and click **Continue**. Provide the required profile information and click **Continue**.
7. Read the Registered User Agreement. Check **Yes, I accept this agreement** and click **Submit**.
8. A screen confirming your enrollment will appear. Click **Get Started** or **My Home**.
9. This product will be added to your Evolve account in the My Content area located on the left-hand side of the Evolve homepage. Click to expand the **Simulations—VMO** heading and then click **Fordney: Insurance Handbook for the Medical Office, Twelfth Edition**.
10. Click **Course Documents** and then click **Simulations—VMO** to access your activities.
11. Your case-sensitive account information will be emailed to you. Please note your account information. If needed, you can request your account information at any time by clicking on **I forgot my login information** on the Evolve homepage.
12. Please bookmark this page (http://evolve.elsevier.com/student) to easily log in and access your *Virtual Medical Office* in the future.

■ SUPPORT INFORMATION

Visit the Evolve Support portal at http://evolvesupport.elsevier.com to access the Evolve Knowledge Base, Downloads, and Support Ticket System. Live Evolve Support is also available 24/7 by calling 1-800-222-9570.

GETTING SET UP

■ TECHNICAL REQUIREMENTS

To use an Evolve online product, you will need access to a computer that is connected to the Internet and equipped with web browser software that supports frames. For optimal performance, it is recommended that you have speakers and use a high-speed Internet connection. Dial-up modems are not recommended for *Virtual Medical Office*.

WINDOWS®

Windows PC
Windows XP, Windows Vista™
Pentium® processor (or equivalent) @ 1 GHz (Recommend 2 GHz or better)
800 x 600 screen size
Thousands of colors
Soundblaster 16 soundcard compatibility
Stereo speakers or headphones
Internet Explorer (IE) version 6.0 or higher
Mozilla Firefox version 2.0 or higher

MACINTOSH®

Mozilla Firefox version 2.0 or higher

■ WEB BROWSERS

Supported web browsers include Microsoft Internet Explorer (IE) version 6.0 or higher and Mozilla Firefox version 2.0 or higher.

Whichever browser you use, the browser preferences must be set to enable cookies and the cache must be set to reload every time.

■ SCREEN SETTINGS

For best results, your computer monitor resolution should be set at a minimum of 800 x 600. The number of colors displayed should be set to "thousands or higher" (High Color or 16 bit) or "millions of colors" (True Color or 24 bit).

WINDOWS

1. From the **Start** menu, select **Settings**, then **Control Panel**.
2. Double-click on the **Display** icon.
3. Click on the **Settings** tab.
4. Under **Screen resolution** use the slider bar to select **800 x 600 pixels**.
5. Access the **Colors** drop-down menu by clicking on the down arrow.
6. Select **High Color (16 bit)** or **True Color (24 bit)**.
7. Click on **Apply**, then **OK**.
8. You may be asked to verify the setting changes. Click **Yes**.
9. You may be asked to restart your computer to accept the changes. Click **Yes**.

MACINTOSH

1. Select the **Monitors** control panel.
2. Select **800 x 600** (or greater) from the **Resolution** area.
3. Select **Thousands** or **Millions** from the **Color Depth** area.

Enable Cookies

Browser	Steps
Internet Explorer (IE) 6.0 or higher	1. Select **Tools → Internet Options**. 2. Select **Privacy** tab. 3. Use the slider (slide down) to **Accept All Cookies**. 4. Click **OK**. -OR- 3. Click the **Advanced** button. 4. Click the check box next to **Override Automatic Cookie Handling**. 5. Click the **Accept** radio buttons under **First-party Cookies** and **Third-party Cookies**. 6. Click **OK**.
Mozilla Firefox 2.0 or higher	1. Select **Tools → Options**. 2. Select the **Privacy** icon. 3. Click to expand Cookies. 4. Select **Allow sites to set cookies**. 5. Click **OK**.

Set Cache to Always Reload a Page

Browser	Steps
Internet Explorer (IE) 6.0 or higher	1. Select **Tools → Internet Options**. 2. Select **General** tab. 3. Go to the **Temporary Internet Files** and click the **Settings** button. 4. Select the radio button for **Every visit to the page** and click **OK** when complete.
Mozilla Firefox 2.0 or higher	1. Select **Tools → Options**. 2. Select the **Privacy** icon. 3. Click to expand Cache. 4. Set the value to "**0**" in the **Use up to: __ MB of disk space for the cache** field. 5. Click **OK**.

Plug-Ins

 Adobe Acrobat Reader—With the free Acrobat Reader software, you can view and print Adobe PDF files. Many Evolve products offer student and instructor manuals, checklists, and more in this format!

Download at: http://www.adobe.com

 Apple QuickTime—Install this to hear word pronunciations, heart and lung sounds, and many other helpful audio clips within Evolve Online Courses!

Download at: http://www.apple.com

 Adobe Flash Player—This player will enhance your viewing of many Evolve web pages, as well as educational short-form to long-form animation within the Evolve Learning System!

Download at: http://www.adobe.com

 Adobe Shockwave Player—Shockwave is best for viewing the many interactive learning activities within Evolve Online Courses!

Download at: http://www.adobe.com

 Microsoft Word Viewer—With this viewer Microsoft Word users can share documents with those who don't have Word, and users without Word can open and view Word documents. Many Evolve products have testbank, student and instructor manuals, and other documents available for down-loading and viewing on your own computer!

Download at: http://www.microsoft.com

Virtual Medical Office Quick Tour

Welcome to *Virtual Medical Office* (VMO), a virtual office setting in which you can work with multiple patient simulations and also learn to access and evaluate the information resources that are essential for providing high-quality medical assistance.

VMO's medical office is called Mountain View Clinic. Once you have signed in to Mountain View Clinic, you can access the Reception area, Exam Room, Laboratory, Office Manager area, and Check-Out area, as well as a separate room for Billing and Coding.

■ BEFORE YOU START

Make sure you have your textbook nearby when you use VMO. You will want to consult topic areas in your textbook frequently while working online and using this Study Guide.

■ HOW TO SIGN IN

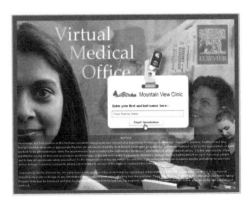

- Access the simulation on the Evolve resource page for your textbook. See the **Getting Started** instructions on page 1 of the Study Guide for information on accessing your Evolve resources.
- Enter your name on the medical assistant identification badge. The name entered here will print out on your performance summary reports.
- Click **Start Simulation**.

- This takes you to the office map screen. Across the top of this screen are photos of patients available for you to follow throughout their office visit.

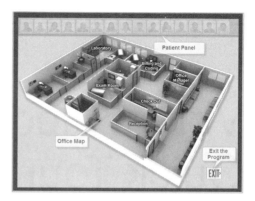

■ PATIENT LIST

1. **Janet Jones (age 50)**—Ms. Jones has sustained an on-the-job injury. She is in pain and impatient. By working with Ms. Jones, students will learn about managing difficult patients, as well as the requirements involved in workers' compensation cases.

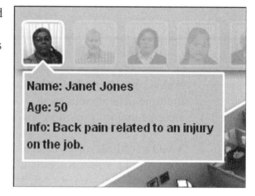

2. **Wilson Metcalf (age 65)**—A Medicare patient, Mr. Metcalf is being seen for multiple symptoms of abdominal pain, nausea, vomiting, and fever. He is seriously ill and might need more specialized care in a hospital setting.

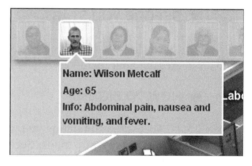

3. **Rhea Davison (age 53)**—An established patient with chronic and multiple symptoms, Ms. Davison does not have medical insurance.

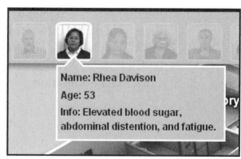

4. **Shaunti Begay (age 15)** — A new patient, Shaunti Begay is a minor who has an appointment for a sports physical. Upon arrival, Shaunti and her family learn that Mountain View Clinic does not participate in their health insurance.

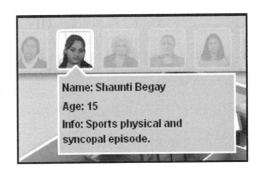

5. **Jean Deere (age 83)** — Accompanied by her son, Ms. Deere is an established Medicare patient being evaluated for memory loss and hearing loss.

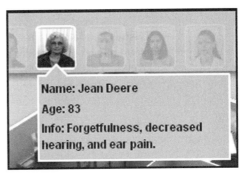

6. **Renee Anderson (age 43)** — Ms. Anderson scheduled her appointment for a routine gynecologic exam but exhibits symptoms that suggest she is a victim of domestic violence.

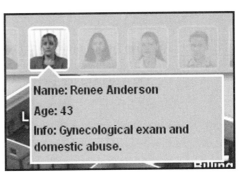

7. **Teresa Hernandez (age 16)** — Teresa is a minor patient who is unaccompanied by a parent for her appointment. She is seeking contraceptive counseling and STD testing.

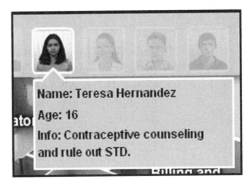

8. **Louise Parlet (age 24)**—Ms. Parlet is an established patient being seen for a pregnancy test and examination. She will also need to be referred to an OB/GYN specialist.

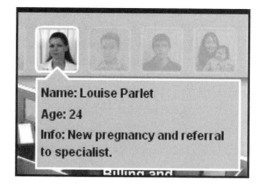

9. **Tristan Tsosie (age 8)**—A minor patient accompanied by his older sister and younger brother, Tristan is having a splint and sutures removed from his injured right arm.

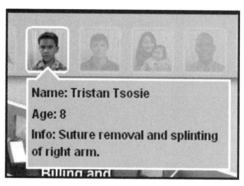

10. **Jose Imero (age 16)**—Jose is a minor patient who is scheduled for an emergency appointment to have the laceration on his foot sutured.

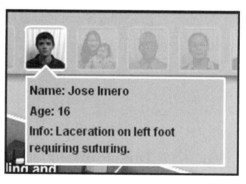

11. **Jade Wong (age 7 months)**—Jade and her parents are new patients to Mountain View Clinic. Jade needs a checkup and updates to her immunizations. Her mother does not speak English.

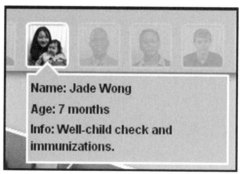

12. **John R. Simmons (age 43)**—Dr. Simmons is a new patient with a history of high blood pressure and recent episodes of blood in his urine.

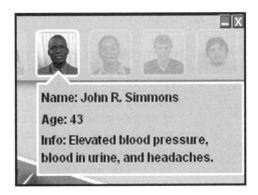

13. **Hu Huang (age 67)**—Mr. Huang developed a severe cough and fever after returning from a recent trip to Asia.

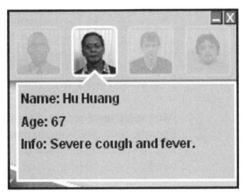

14. **Kevin McKinzie (age 18)**—Mr. McKinzie has made an appointment because of his nausea and vomiting. He is insured through the restaurant where he works.

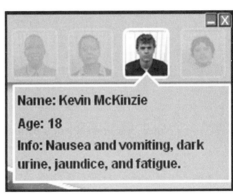

15. **Jesus Santo (age 32)**—Mr. Santo has been brought to the office as a walk-in appointment by his employer for leg pain and a fever. He has no insurance or identification, but his employer has offered to pay for the visit.

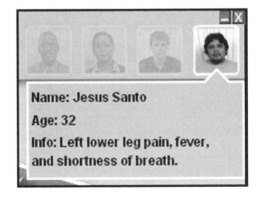

■ BASIC NAVIGATION

HOW TO SELECT A PATIENT

The list of patients is located across the top of the office map screen. Pointing your cursor at the various patients will highlight their photo and reveal their name, age, and medical problem (see examples in the illustrations on the previous pages). When you click on the patient you wish to review, a larger photo and description will appear in the lower left corner of the screen.

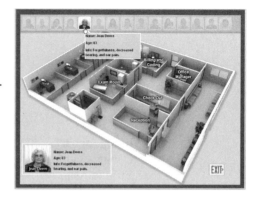

HOW TO SELECT A ROOM

After selecting a patient, use your cursor to highlight the room you want to enter. The active room will be shaded blue on the map. Click to enter the room.

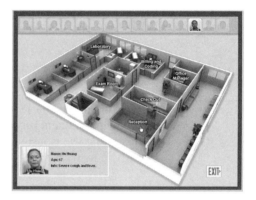

Note: You **must** select a patient before you are allowed access to any room.

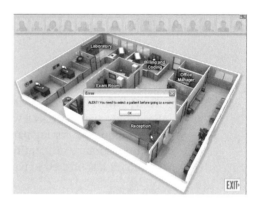

HOW TO LEAVE A ROOM

When you are finished working in a room, you can leave by clicking the exit arrow found at the bottom right corner of the screen.

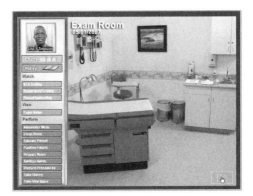

Leaving a room will automatically take you to the Summary Menu.

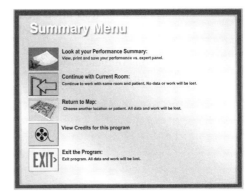

From the Summary Menu, you can choose to:

- **Look at Your Performance Summary**

  In each room there are interactive wizards or tasks that can be completed. The Performance Summary lets you compare your answers with those of the experts.

- **Continue with Current Room**

  This takes you back to the last room in which you worked. This option is not available if you have already reviewed your Performance Summary.

- **Return to Map**

  This reopens the office map for you to select another room and/or another patient.

- **View Credits for This Program**

  This provides a complete listing of software developers, publisher, and authors.

- **Exit the Program**

  This closes the *Virtual Medical Office* software. You will need to sign in again before you can use the program.

Note: If you choose to return to the office map, VMO alerts you that all unsaved room data will be lost. This means that any tasks completed in that room will be reset. Choose **Yes** to continue to the office map or **No** to return to the Summary Menu, where you can choose to continue working in the room or look at your Performance Summary.

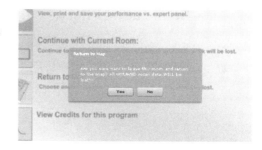

HOW TO USE THE PERFORMANCE SUMMARY

If you completed any of the interactive wizards in a room, you can compare your answers with those of the experts by accessing your Performance Summary. This feature can be accessed after working in the Reception area, Exam Room, Laboratory, and Check Out area. The Performance Summary is not a grading tool, although it is valuable for self-assessment and review.

From the Summary Menu, click on **Look at Your Performance Summary**.

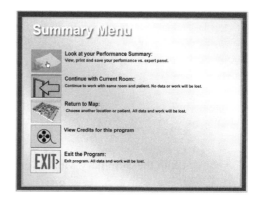

The complete list of tasks associated with the active room will appear with two columns showing the results of your choices. Your answers will appear in the column labeled **Your Performance**, and the answers chosen by the expert will appear in the **Expert's Performance** column. A check mark in both columns for a given task indicates that your answer matched the expert's answer. The Performance Summary can be saved to your computer or disk by clicking on the disk icon at the upper right side of the screen. The saved file can be printed or e-mailed to your instructor. A hard copy can also be printed without saving by clicking on the printer icon at the upper right corner of the screen.

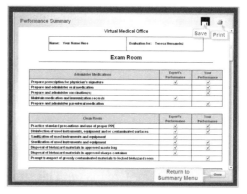

■ ROOM DESCRIPTIONS

All rooms can be entered at any time and in any order. You can follow a patient's visit from Reception to Check Out, or you can choose to observe patients at any point in their care. Below is a description of the information and activities that can be found in various rooms.

ALL ROOMS

- You can access the patient's medical record (Charts) and the office Policy Manual in all rooms.
- Each room has a sidebar Room Menu, from which you can choose to view documents, perform tasks, and watch videos.

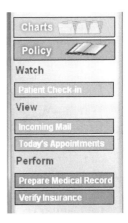

- The Reception area, Exam Room, and Check Out areas all feature videos in which you can watch the medical assistant interact with other Mountain View Clinic personnel and patients. Within the video screen you have a variety of options for navigating. Hover your cursor over the controls and status bar along the bottom of the video screen to reveal how each functions. By clicking various controls, you can play the video, pause it, forward or rewind using the scroll bar, and adjust the volume. Pressing the square stop button will stop the video and return the scroll bar to the beginning. Close the video screen by clicking on the **X** in the upper right corner of the screen.

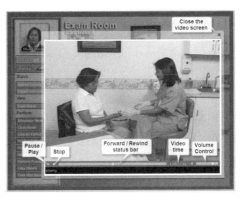

- Almost all rooms have **View** and **Perform** options on the Room Menu (*Note:* The Billing and Coding area does not have any Perform functions). These tasks can be completed either by clicking on the task description in the Room Menu or by clicking on the corresponding object in the room area. (For example, during an exercise, if you are required to perform the task of sanitizing your hands, the instructions may be worded as "Click on **Sanitize Hands** under Perform on the Room Menu," or you may simply be asked to "Click on the **Sink**." Both routes take you to the same task.) As you move your cursor over each item connected to one of the tasks on the View or Perform menu, both the object and the corresponding task in the Room Menu will highlight and become active. (*Note:* All corresponding pairs of instruction cues are listed in the individual room descriptions on the following pages.)

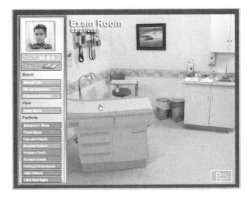

RECEPTION

In the Reception area, you can choose:

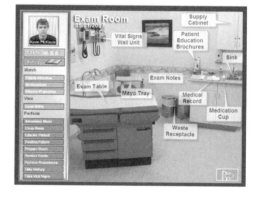

- **Charts**—Look at the patient's chart. *Note:* For new patients, there will be no information available in the chart at this time, although you do have the option of assembling a new medical record.
- **Policy**—Open the office Policy Manual and review the established administrative, clinical, and laboratory policies for Mountain View Clinic. Within the Policy Manual you will also find the Coding and Billing Manual.
- **Watch**—Watch a video of the patient's arrival. Each patient is shown checking in at the front desk so that you can observe the procedures typically performed by the receptionist and consider some of the various problems that might arise.
- **View**—Look at the Incoming Mail for the day by clicking on the stack of letters located on the **Stackable Trays** on the Reception desk. Review Today's Appointments by clicking on the **Computer** on the Reception desk to open up the day's schedule.
- **Perform**—Perform tasks at the Reception desk that are part of an administrative medical assistant's duties. Practice how to Prepare a Medical Record for a patient by clicking on the **Medical Record** file folder on the Reception desk. Verify Insurance for a patient by clicking on the **Insurance Card** on the counter at the Reception desk window.

EXAM ROOM

- **Charts** and **Policy**—Access the patient's chart and the office Policy Manual.
- **Watch**—View videos of different parts of the patient's exam. Observe the actions of the medical assistants in the videos and critique the competencies demonstrated.
- **View**—Review the physician's documented findings for the current visit in the Exam Notes. These notes are added to the full Progress Notes in the patient's chart as the patient continues on to Check Out. This can be accessed by clicking on the **Exam Notes** on the Exam Room counter.
- **Perform**—Perform multiple tasks that are required of a clinical medical assistant, such as preparing the room for the exam, taking vital signs and patient history, and properly positioning the patient for an exam. For each task listed under Perform on the Room Menu (cues on the left below), a corresponding object in the room area (cues on the right below) can also be clicked to access and perform the task:
  - **Administer Meds = Medication Cup**
  - **Clean Room = Waste Receptacles**
  - **Educate Patient = Patient Education Brochures**
  - **Position Patient = Exam Table**
  - **Prepare Room = Supply Cabinet**
  - **Sanitize Hands = Sink**
  - **Perform Procedures = Mayo Tray**
  - **Take History = Medical Record**
  - **Take Vital Signs = Vital Signs Wall Unit**

LABORATORY

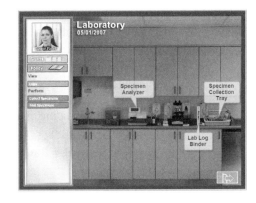

- **Charts** and **Policy**—Access the patient's chart and the office Policy Manual.
- **View**—View the laboratory's log of specimens sent out for testing. Opportunities to practice filling out laboratory logs are included in the Study Guide exercises. This can be accessed by clicking on the **Lab Log Binder** on the Laboratory counter.
- **Perform**—Perform specific tasks as needed in the laboratory, such as collecting and testing specimens. These interactive wizards walk you through the steps for collecting and testing specimens ordered by the physician as part of the patient's exam. Access the Collect Specimens function by clicking on the **Specimen Collection Tray** on the counter. Complete the Test Specimens task by clicking on the **Specimen Analyzer**, also on the laboratory counter.

CHECK OUT

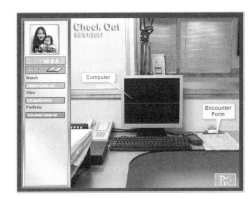

- **Charts** and **Policy**—Access the patient's chart and the office Policy Manual.
- **Watch**—Watch a video of the patient checking out of the office at the end of the visit. Observe the administrative medical assistants as they schedule follow-up appointments, accept payments, and manage the various duties and problems that may arise.
- **View**—The Encounter Form for each patient's visit can be accessed by clicking on the **Encounter Form** on the clipboard on the Check Out desk.
- **Perform**—Certain patients will require a return visit to the office. Schedule their follow-up appointments as needed by clicking on the **Computer** on the Check Out desk.

BILLING AND CODING

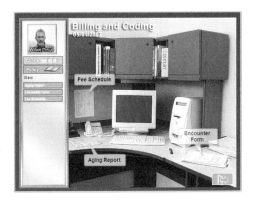

- **Charts** and **Policy**—Access the patient's chart and the office Policy Manual.
- **View**—Review the outstanding balances on various patient accounts and assess when to implement different collection techniques by clicking on the **Aging Report** on the left side of the Billing and Coding desk. Use the patient's **Encounter Form** on the right side of the desk to determine whether the proper procedures were followed to ensure accurate billing and coding. The office's **Fee Schedule** (on the wall to the left of the computer) is used to calculate the proper charges for the patient's visit.

OFFICE MANAGER

- **Policy**—View the office Policy Manual. Note that patient charts are not available from the Office Manager area.
- **View**—A variety of financial and administrative documents are available for viewing in the Office Manager area to practice managing office finances. Corresponding clues are listed below (menu terms on left; object cues on right):
  - **Bank Statement = Bank Statement** green file folder
  - **Day Sheet = Day Sheet** to the right of the computer keyboard

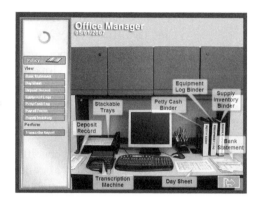

  - **Deposit Record = Deposit Record** to the left of the **Transcription Machine**
  - **Equipment Logs = Equipment Log Binder**
  - **Petty Cash Log = Petty Cash Binder**
  - **Payroll Forms** = located in the **Stackable Trays**
  - **Supply Inventory = Supply Inventory Binder**
- **Perform**—A recorded medical report is included for transcription practice with full player controls. This can be accessed by clicking on the Transcription Machine to the left of the computer keyboard.

■ EMBEDDED ERRORS

The individual lessons and patient scenarios associated with the *Virtual Medical Office* program were designed to stimulate critical thinking and analytical skills and to help develop the competencies you will be tested on as part of your course work. Thus deliberate errors have been embedded into each of the 15 patient scenarios and in the Billing and Coding and Office Manager activities. Many of the exercises in the Study Guide draw attention to these errors so that you can learn to recognize when and why a correction needs to be made, as well as how to correct it. Other errors have not been specifically addressed, and you may discover them as you work through the various rooms and tasks. These errors, when found, provide great learning opportunities to further develop the essential critical thinking and decision-making skills needed for professional work in the clinical office.

The following icons are used throughout the Study Guide to help you quickly identify particular activities and assignments:

 Reading Assignment—tells you which textbook chapter(s) you should read before starting each lesson

 Writing Activity—certain activities focus on written responses such as filling out forms or completing documentation

 Online Activity—marks the beginning of an activity that uses the *Virtual Medical Office* simulation software

 Online Instructions—indicates the steps to follow as you navigate through the software

 Reference—indicates questions and activities that require you to consult your textbook

 Time—indicates the approximate amount of time needed to complete the exercise

Virtual Medical Office Detailed Tour

If you wish to understand the capabilities of *Virtual Medical Office* more thoroughly, take a detailed tour by completing the following exercises. During this tour, we will work with a specific patient to introduce you to all the different components and learning opportunities available within the VMO software for the Medical Insurance/Billing & Coding student.

Exercise 1

Online Activity—Role of an Insurance Billing Specialist

45 minutes

- Sign in to Mountain View Clinic and select **Shaunti Begay** from the patient list. Highlight the **Reception** area and click to enter. Remember, you cannot enter any of the rooms on the map until a patient is selected.

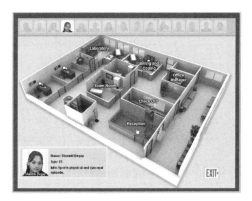

- You are now at the **Reception** desk, where Shaunti Begay will check in for her appointments. In this room you can watch the Check-In video for important information about her visit and review her insurance information.

- From the Room Menu under the Watch heading, select **Patient Check-In** and watch the video of Shaunti checking in for her appointment. You can use the video controls to pause, rewind, fast-forward, and adjust the volume as you watch.

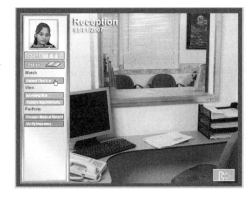

1. What information about Shaunti Begay and her visit were you able to gather from the video? Select all that apply from the list below.

   _____ Shaunti is a new patient at the practice.

   _____ Shaunti is an established patient at the practice.

   _____ Shaunti has an appointment with Dr. Hayler.

   _____ Shaunti is being seen for a sports physical examination.

   _____ Shaunti's father works on Fifth Avenue.

➤ • When you are finished, click on the **X** at the top right of the video screen to close the video and return to the Reception desk.

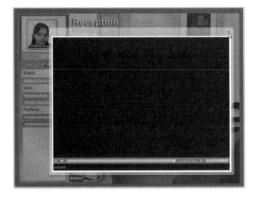

• To confirm Shaunti's appointment, click on the **Computer** to view Today's Appointments. This will open Mountain View Clinic's appointment schedule for the day's visits. *Note:* The virtual date for the Mountain View Clinic is May 1, 2007. Use the scroll bar to view both morning and afternoon appointments.

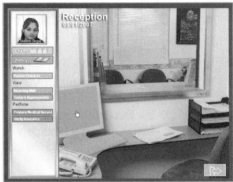

2. Which provider is Shaunti scheduled to see?
   a. Dr. Hayler
   b. Dr. Meyer

3. What time is Shaunti's appointment scheduled for?

4. Take a moment to skim over the rest of today's appointments. Of the other patients being seen today, which one has SMO insurance?

- Click **Finish** to return to the Reception desk. According to the video you watched, a problem has developed with Shaunti's insurance. Click on the **Insurance Card** on the counter to verify her insurance.

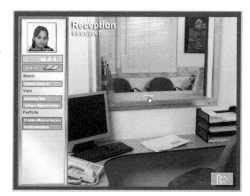

- You are instructed to choose an appropriate question to ask Shaunti. Selecting the correct question depends on whether she is a new or an established patient. Because this is Shaunti's first visit to the office, she is a new patient. Thus the second question choice does not apply because no records are currently on file that need to be changed or updated. Click the **Ask** button next to "Do you have insurance?"

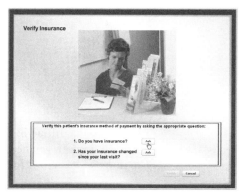

- Next, you will be asked to follow through on the information provided by the patient to complete her insurance verification. If you need more information about the patient's insurance, you can use the buttons at the bottom left of the screen to view her insurance card or her completed Patient Information Form. Click on **Insurance Card(s)** to view the back and front of Shaunti's insurance card.

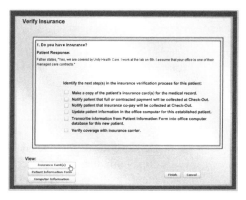

5. Shaunti's insurance card was issued by:
   a. Blue Cross/Blue Shield.
   b. Medicaid.
   c. Unity Health Care.

6. The Group Number indicated on Shaunti's insurance card is:
   a. 4B22.
   b. 6144.
   c. M238458888.
   d. 86756.

7. The issue date on Shaunti's insurance card is:
   a. May 1, 2007.
   b. April 1, 2001.

- Click the **Back** button to return to the Verify Insurance screen. (*Note:* If you click **Finish**, you will be taken back to the Reception desk and you will not be able to return to the Verify Insurance task unless you exit to the office map and reenter the Reception desk.)

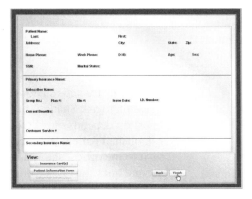

- Many physicians' offices now use computers to track their patients' personal and medical information. Click on the **Computer Information** button on the lower left of the screen to see a typical screen used for entering this information.

8. Below, practice filling in Shaunti's information for the first section of the screen. You can locate all the data you need to complete this screen by clicking to view the **Insurance Card(s)** and **Patient information Form** at the lower left side of your screen.

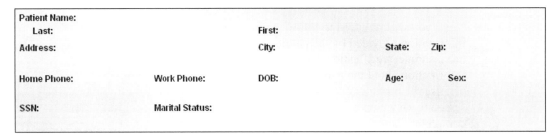

- Because the office does not accept the Begays' insurance plan, the staff cannot accept the copay amount and must collect the full amount due when Shaunti checks out. Make sure you identify all the steps necessary to finish verifying her insurance. The next steps are to:
  - Make a copy of the insurance cards for the medical record.
  - Notify Shaunti's parents that full payment will be expected at the end of the visit.
  - Enter the new patient information in the computer.
  - Verify coverage with the insurance carrier.

- Click on **Finish** to return to the Reception desk.

- Before we continue, look at the Verify Insurance button on the Room Menu. Has anything changed? Note that each time you complete a task under the Perform menu in any room, the corresponding menu selection bar lightens and a check mark appears next to the task. Because you have completed this task (Verify Insurance), you will not be able to access the task again unless you exit the room, return to the office map, and select this room again. (*Note:* The tasks on the Room Menu do not necessarily appear in the order in which they should be completed.)

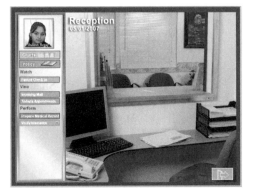

- In the video, Kristin, the receptionist, offered the Begays a copy of the office's policies. Click on the **Policy** button to review Mountain View Clinic's policies.

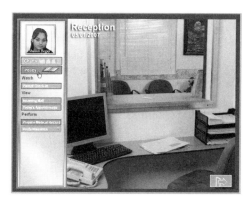

- You have several options for searching and navigating the Policy Manual. You can type specific keywords in the search bar, use the Table of Contents menu on the left to browse through particular sections, use the scroll bar and arrows on the right side of the screen, or jump to a specific page by using the page number box or the page-turn arrows.

- The policy on accepted insurance carriers is located on page 33 of the Policy Manual. Using any of the methods described above will take you to the correct location. Try all four routes for practice:

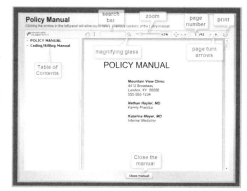

  - Type the word *insurance* in the search bar and click on the magnifying glass or press Enter on your keyboard. This will search the Policy Manual for that specific term. You will need to continue to click on the magnifying glass until you locate the section of the Policy Manual you need. (***Remember:*** The magnifying glass is for finding, not for zooming in. To enlarge text for easier reading, use the zoom bar to the right of the magnifying glass.)
  - Use the scroll bar and arrows to flip to the correct page of the Policy Manual.
  - Type "33" in the page number box and press Enter on your keyboard.
  - Expand the Table of Contents until you find the correct area. Click on the relevant heading to go there. (***Note:*** Mountain View Clinic's policy on accepted insurance carriers is located in the Billing and Coding Manual under the Financial Policy section.)

9. Which of the following are accepted insurance carriers at Mountain View Clinic? Select all that apply.

   _____ State Health Insurance

   _____ Unity Health Care

   _____ Oasis Health

   _____ Star Insurance

   _____ Local Supplement Health Group

   _____ Medicaid

   _____ Mutual Health Insurance Company

   _____ Midwestern HMO

   _____ Workers' Compensation

- Click **Close Manual** at the bottom of the screen to return to the Reception desk.
- Click on **Charts** button at the top of the Room Menu. Because Shaunti is a new patient, there are no records yet in her chart. As Shaunti progresses through her visit, forms and charts will be added to her medical record.

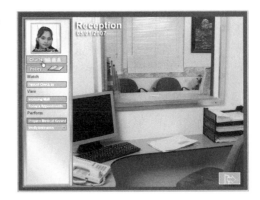

- Click on **Close Chart** to return to the Reception desk.

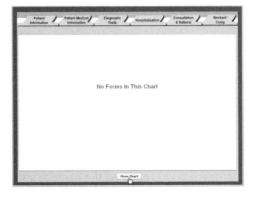

- Take a moment to look through the day's mail. Click on the pile of letters in the **Stackable Trays** on the right side of the Reception desk. The screen opens to reveal a letter to Dr. Meyer from Dr. William Neurg.

- To see the rest of the day's mail, use the directional arrows at the top of the screen or click on the number of the piece of mail you want to review. Click to view each piece of the **Incoming Mail**.

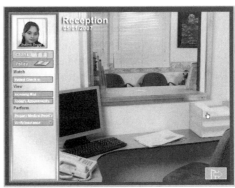

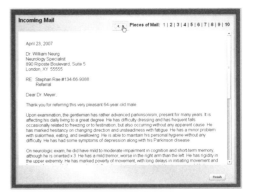

10. How many total pieces of mail are there to be reviewed?

11. How many checks were received in the mail?

• Click on **Finish** to return to Reception. It is time to leave the room and follow Shaunti to the Exam Room. Click on the exit arrow in the lower right corner of the screen to leave the Reception desk.

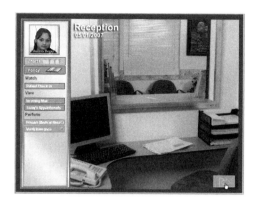

• At the Summary Menu screen, click on **Return to Map** to follow Shaunti's progress in the Exam Room.

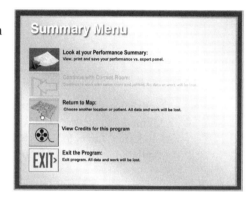

• Each time you return to the Office Map, *Virtual Medical Office* alerts you that all unsaved room data will be lost. This means any tasks completed, such as verifying insurance, will be reset. If you choose No, you will be returned to the Summary Menu, where you can continue working in the current room, review your Performance Summary, or exit the program. For your current assignment, click **Yes** to return to the Office Map.

• You are now ready to follow Shaunti to the Exam Room.

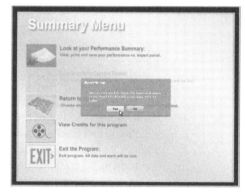

Exercise 2

 Online Activity—Exam Room

 10 minutes

- Shaunti Begay will remain as your patient unless you exit the VMO software or select another patient. Keep Shaunti as your patient for this exercise. Use your mouse to highlight the Exam Room on the office map and click to enter.

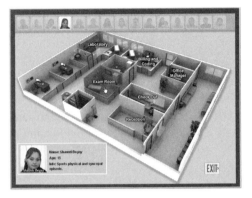

- Both Shaunti's chart and the office Policy Manual can be accessed within the room. Click on **Charts** to see what information is available in the Exam Room.

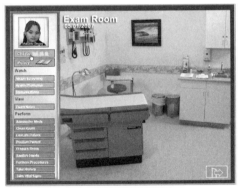

- The chart opens to Shaunti's Patient Information Form. Across the top of the chart are tabs under which you can find additional information about Shaunti's visit. As you click on each tab, a drop-down menu appears, listing all the available information under that tab.

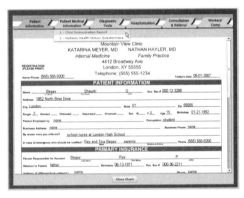

1. Click on the **Patient Information** tab. What documentation is included under this tab?

    (1)

    (2)

    (3)

    (4)

    (5)

2. Which of the following tabs do not currently have any forms? Select all that apply.

_____ Patient Information

_____ Patient Medical Information

_____ Diagnostic Tests

_____ Hospitalizations

_____ Consultation & Referral

_____ Workers' Comp

 • Click **Close Chart** at the bottom of the screen to return to the Exam Room.
• Click on the **Exam Notes** clipboard to view Shaunti's Exam Notes as summarized from her Progress Notes by the physician.

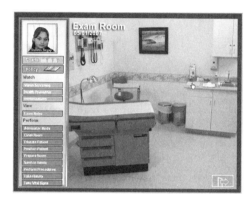

3. Where will the ECG testing for Shaunti be performed?
   a. At Shaunti's home
   b. At Mountain View Clinic
   c. At the hospital

4. Indicate whether the following statement is true or false.

_____ The Health Assessment for Teens (HEADSS) finds Shaunti to be an underactive teenager.

• Click the **Finish** button to return to the Exam Room. Click on the exit arrow at the bottom right of the screen to exit the room. On the Summary Menu, click **Return to Map**. Again, a pop-up message will inform you that all data will be lost. Click **Yes** to return to the office map and continue with Shaunti to the Check Out area.

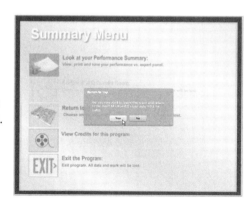

Exercise 3

 Online Activity—Check Out Area

 30 minutes

- Shaunti and her family are ready to proceed to Mountain View Clinic's Check Out area, where they will pay for Shaunti's visit and collect any information they might need for after they leave.
- On the office map, click on **Check Out**.

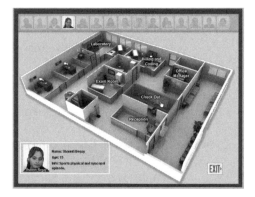

- Once again, Shaunti's chart and the office Policy Manual are both accessible. Click on **Charts** to review the documents added to Shaunti's medical record since she left the Exam Room.

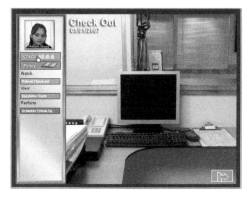

1. Click on all tabs at the top of Shaunti's chart to see what forms are included under each. Which of the tabs listed below still have no forms in them? Select all that apply.

_____ Patient Information

_____ Patient Medical Information

_____ Diagnostic Tests

_____ Hospitalization

_____ Consultation and Referral

_____ Workers' Comp

- Click on the **Patient Medical Information** tab, and from the drop-down menu, select **2-Progress Notes**. Scroll through the Progress Notes until you reach the last entry at 3:15 p.m.

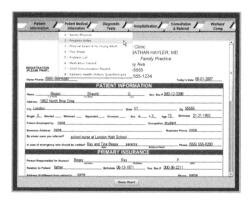

2. Indicate whether the following statement is true or false.

_____ According to the 3:15 p.m. entry in the Progress Notes, Shaunti will be scheduled to see a dermatologist who takes her insurance, Unity Health Plan.

- Click on the **Consultation & Referral** tab, and select **1-Referral Form** from the drop-down menu.
- Read through the form and note the headings of each section on the form. These sections provide all the basic information the clinic will need to arrange Shaunti's appointment, including her insurance information and the reason for the referral.

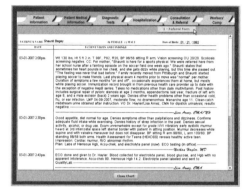

3. What condition is listed as the reason for the referral?

4. What ICD-9 diagnosis codes are listed on the referral form to indicate medical necessity of this referral to the Braeburn Cardiology Clinic?

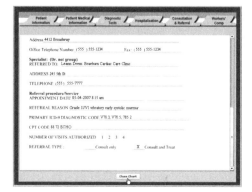

- Click **Close Chart** at the bottom of the screen to return to the Check Out area.

- On the room menu, click on **Patient Check-Out** under the Watch heading and watch the video of Shaunti's check-out.
- Click the **X** at the top right of the screen to close the video.

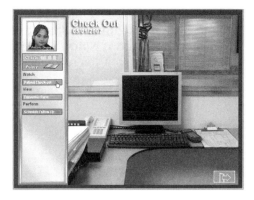

5. In this video, Mr. Begay expresses his surprise at:
   a. how much time they have had to wait for an appointment.
   b. the number of laboratory tests that the physician ordered.
   c. how quickly they are able to get an appointment with the referring provider.
   d. the amount of money due for Shaunti's examination.

6. What is offered to Mr. Begay that would provide an explanation of the charge for every services provided?

- Click on the **Encounter Form** clipboard to the right of the computer.
- Scroll through the Encounter Form and note what items were checked off for Shaunti's visit.

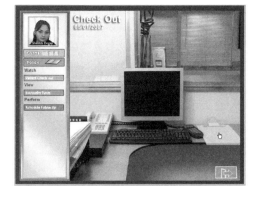

7. What are the total charges for Shaunti's visit?

8. How much did Mr. Begay pay at check-out?

9. What is the balance remaining for this visit?

- Click **Finish** to return to the Check Out area.
- Click on the **Computer** to schedule Shaunti for her follow-up appointment.

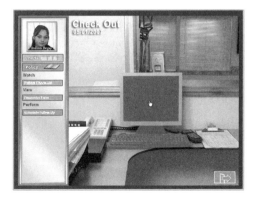

- Several steps are listed that might need to be taken to schedule a follow-up appointment for a patient. Depending on what the patient needs, you might need to select a few of these steps or you might need to select only one.

- For Shaunti, check the boxes next to **Schedule a referral to specialist**, and **Receive co-pay/ payment**. Click **Finish** to return to Check Out.

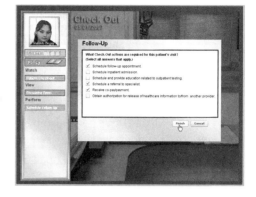

- You have completed the steps necessary for Shaunti's Check Out. Click on the exit arrow to leave the room and go to the Summary Menu.

- On the Summary Menu, click **Return to Map**. The pop-up message will inform you that all data will be lost. Click **Yes** to return to the office map and continue with Shaunti in the Billing and Coding area.

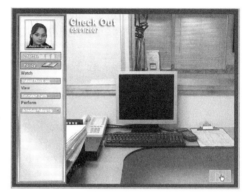

Exercise 4

Online Activity—Billing and Coding

45 minutes

- Although Shaunti and her family have checked out from their appointment and have left the office, more needs to be done to process Shaunti's visit to the Mountain View Clinic.

- On the office map, click on **Billing and Coding**.

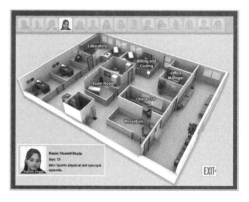

• Because we still have Shaunti selected as an active patient, her chart remains accessible in the Billing and Coding area along with the office Policy Manual. As you saw in other rooms, the chart has been updated and now contains the most current documentation. This documentation now includes not only what occurred during Shaunti's visit but also the records from her previous physician.

• Click on **Charts** to open Shaunti's medical record.

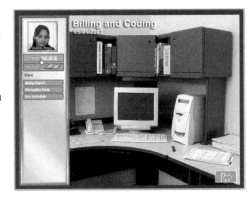

1. Click on all tabs at the top of the chart and identify which of the tabs listed below have no forms or information in them. Select all that apply.

_____ Patient Information

_____ Patient Medical Information

_____ Diagnostic Tests

_____ Hospitalization

_____ Consultation and Referral

_____ Workers' Comp

→ • Click on the **Hospitalization** tab and select **1-Operative Report**.

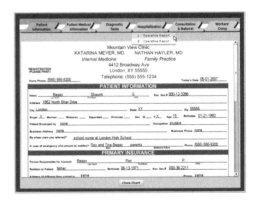

2. What is the encounter date listed on the report?

3. Read through the report. How old was Shaunti when this operation occurred?

4. What is the condition that Shaunti was being treated for?

5. What is the name of the operative procedure that was performed?

- Next, click on the **Consultation & Referral** tab and select **2-Office Notes** from the drop-down menu.

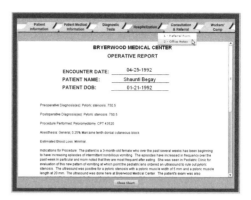

6. What is the encounter date on this report?

7. What is the name of the facility that issued this report?

8. Read through the report. How old was Shaunti at the time of this visit?

9. Why was Shaunti brought to the clinic to be seen on this date?

10. What is the name of the provider that treated Shaunti?

- Click on the **Patient Information** tab and select **1-Patient Information Form**.

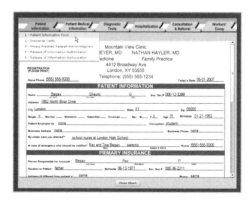

11. Medical Insurance and Billing & Coding students will be given exercises in filling out the CMS-1500 claim form. Using the information found on Shaunti's Patient Information Form, fill in the top portion of the CMS-1500 form below (Blocks 2, 3, 5, 6, and 8). *Hint:* Blocks 2 and 5 must be entered in ALL CAPS with no punctuation.

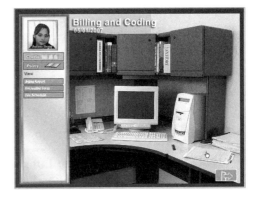

- Click **Close Chart** to return to the Billing and Coding area.
- A main source of information for Billing and Coding is the Encounter Form. Click on the **Encounter Form** file to the right of the computer to review the list of charges for Shaunti's visit.

12. According to the Encounter Form, what type of insurance does Shaunti's family have?
    a. Private
    b. BCBS
    c. Medicare
    d. Medicaid
    e. HMO
    f. Tricare

13. All of the services that were provided to Shaunti are listed on the Encounter Form. List the nine services that were provided.

(1)

(2)

(3)

(4)

(5)

(6)

(7)

(8)

(9)

- Click **Finish** to return to the Billing and Coding area.

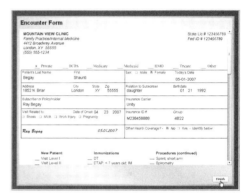

- To calculate charges on the Encounter Form, you need to know what the office fee is for each service. Click on the **Fee Schedule** on the wall above the telephone to view the full list of services and charges.

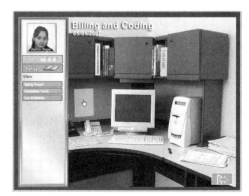

14. Determine the amount due for each of the nine services you listed in question 13 and itemize them below.

(1)

(2)

(3)

(4)

(5)

(6)

(7)

(8)

(9)

➡ • Click **Finish** to return to the Billing and Coding area.

• The Aging Report is a tool used to keep track of patient accounts by recording the date and amount of the bill, as well as the date and amount of payment. The Aging Report also identifies balances that are becoming overdue, usually in increments of 30 days.

• Click on the **Aging Report** blue file to the left of the computer to view the current patient balances.

15. What are the starting and ending dates for this Aging Report?

Starting Date: Ending Date:

16. The first patient on the report is Jacob Abraham. His service (99201) was billed at the rate

of _____.

17. The report indicates that Mr. Abraham made a payment of _____ on his account.

18. The date Mr. Abraham made the cash payment was _____.

19. What is the balance due by Mr. Abraham?

20. What is the age of the balance that Mr. Abraham owes?
    a. 31-60 days old
    b. 61-90 days old
    c. 91-120 days old
    d. Over 120 days old

→ • Scroll to the bottom of the Aging Report.

21. The total amount of the accounts receivable for both providers is _____.

22. Of the entire accounts receivable for both providers, what percentage is over 120 days old?

→ • Click **Finish** to return to the Billing and Coding area.

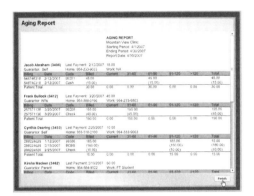

• You have now finished working in the Billing and Coding area. Click on the exit arrow to leave the room and go the Summary Menu.

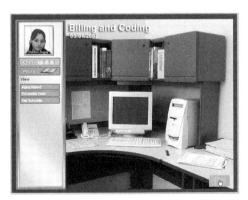

- Click **Exit the Program**. A pop-up message will inform you that all data will be lost. Click **Yes** to close the program.

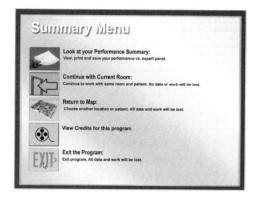

Congratulations! You have completed the *Virtual Medical Office* tours, which were designed to introduce you to the software and the various components you will be working with throughout this learning experience.

Role of an Insurance Billing Specialist

 Reading Assignment: Chapter 1—Role of an Insurance Billing Specialist

Patient: Wilson Metcalf

Room: Reception

Objectives:

- Demonstrate an understanding of the role of an insurance billing specialist.
- Recognize the importance of the organization's office policies as a resource in reducing potential violations in medical law, liability, or ethical issues.
- Identify potential liabilities and ethical issues occurring in the medical office.
- Identify breaches of medical ethics and etiquette and determine a more appropriate method of handling the situation.
- Demonstrate an understanding of the importance of the health insurance professional to be a team player within the medical office.

Exercise 1

 Online Activity—Role of an Insurance Billing Specialist

20 minutes

- Sign in to Mountain View Clinic.
- Select **Wilson Metcalf** from the patient list.
- Click on **Reception**.
- Click on **Policy** to open the office Policy Manual.
- Type "job description" in the search bar and click once on the magnifying glass.
- Read the job descriptions for all the office medical assisting positions.

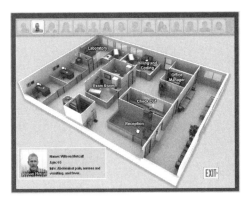

1. Based on what you have read in the textbook chapter and in the Policy Manual, why is it important for the insurance billing specialist to be familiar with all aspects of the medical office? Check all that apply.

   _____ The insurance billing specialist's primary goal is to assist in the revenue cycle and the flow of information from all areas that affect payment of service.

   _____ The insurance billing specialist will need to work well with other clinical and business office personnel to ensure a strong billing cycle and enhanced reimbursement for service provided.

   _____ The insurance billing specialist will need to ensure that all information submitted to the insurance carrier is correct to avoid payment delays.

   _____ The insurance billing specialist may be the next in line for another position within the practice.

2. An individual who does billing and completes insurance claims must have many skills. Based on the job descriptions provided in the textbook and in the office Policy Manual, identify five or six specific skills in which you will need to become extremely proficient for the position of entry-level insurance billing specialist.

3. Why is it important for the insurance billing specialist to have knowledge of compliance issues and medicolegal rules and regulations of various insurance programs?

4. Why is it important for the insurance billing specialist to be a team player?

5. The Policy Manual states "teamwork is the foundation of successful employment in this office" and suggests that employees share responsibilities. Assuming you have been hired as the insurance billing specialist, what other roles and responsibilities might you be expected to perform?

 • Keep the Policy Manual open and continue to the next exercise.

Exercise 2

 ### Online Activity—Medical Law and General Liability

 30 minutes

It is the insurance billing specialist's responsibility to conduct business in a legal and ethical manner. The health insurance professional must be knowledgeable in the areas of medical law and liability that will affect them. An organization's Policy Manual can serve as a foundation in protecting the health insurance professional from lawsuits or violations of health care laws and regulations. The first step that new employees should take is to thoroughly familiarize themselves with their organization's Policy Manual.

Note: Keep in mind that office policies vary from one practice to the next.

 • Click on **Policy Manual** in the Table of Contents in the left pane on your screen.
• Read the Mountain View Clinic Policy Manual in its entirety. Move through the pages by using the scroll bar on the right side of the manual or the arrow buttons at the top right side of the page. You will be using the information from this manual as you proceed through all exercises in the Virtual Medical Office workbook. If needed, you can print the Mountain View Clinic Policy Manual using the button in the upper right corner.
• Keep the Policy Manual open to answer the following questions.

1. The purposes of Mountain View Clinic's Policy Manual include all of the following except:
   a. documenting standards of conduct.
   b. ensuring compliance with all health care laws and regulations.
   c. providing the health insurance professional with health care laws.
   d. identifying what behavior is expected of employees.

2. According to the job description in Mountain View Clinic's Policy Manual, it is the health insurance professional's responsibility to:
   a. adhere to federal guidelines regarding third-party reimbursement.
   b. adhere to state guidelines regarding third-party reimbursement.
   c. adhere to third-party payer policies regarding reimbursement.
   d. adhere to federal, state, and third-party payer policies regarding third-party reimbursement.

3. According to the job description in Mountain View Clinic's Policy Manual, to avoid violation of health care fraud or abuse, the health insurance professional should report the ICD-9 and CPT codes that are:
   a. assigned by the provider on the Encounter Form.
   b. assigned by the provider on the Encounter Form after verifying that they are supported in the documentation.
   c. most likely to result in the claim being paid.
   d. most frequently used.

4. Indicate whether the following statement is true or false.

   _____ The health insurance professional at Mountain View Clinic may perform the duties of a registered or licensed practical nurse if requested to do so by the physician.

5. Assume that you are a health insurance professional working at Mountain View Clinic. A patient in the waiting room begins to show signs of a medical crisis. What should you do?
   a. Don't get involved; it is not your responsibility since you are a health insurance professional.
   b. Request additional help by saying, "Please get the red folder!"
   c. Request additional help by saying, "Is there a doctor in the house?"
   d. Clear the waiting room.

6. Occasionally, during a phone conversation with a patient regarding a bill, the health insurance professional at Mountain View Clinic may be asked a medical question. The health insurance professional:
   a. may give advice based on his or her experience in the office.
   b. may give advice based on what is written in the patient's record.
   c. may give advice based on a note left by the physician.
   d. may never give advice on the telephone.

7. You are a health insurance professional at Mountain View Clinic. A patient contacts you, identifying himself as a physician-colleague who is requesting a professional courtesy. You should:
   a. write off this patient's entire bill immediately.
   b. explain to the patient that this could be a violation of the Medicare Anti-Kickback statute and you are therefore unable to honor the request.
   c. refuse to honor the request and hang up the phone immediately.
   d. process this as an "insurance only" billing.

8. When is the discounting of fees allowed at Mountain View Clinic?
   a. Routinely, for any patient you think deserves it
   b. For all patients over 65 who have Medicare
   c. Never
   d. Only for those services that are not covered by any health insurance plan and that will not be submitted to an insurance carrier for payment

9. According to Mountain View Clinic's Policy Manual, when may you, as the health insurance professional, submit a claim that is known to contain inaccurate information?
   a. When the provider tells you to submit it with inaccurate information
   b. When the charge ticket has been completed with that same inaccurate information
   c. When the receptionist co-signs the charge slip containing the inaccurate information
   d. When you have obtained guidance from the compliance leader(s) or the office administrator(s) and the resolution has been documented in writing

10. As the health insurance professional at Mountain View Clinic, if you are unsure of the rules or regulations related to any situation you are confronted with, you should:
    a. proceed with caution.
    b. stop, reconsider the situation, use your best judgment, and document it.
    c. take the advice of a co-worker with more experience.
    d. obtain guidance from the billing manager, compliance officer, or office administrator.

11. Based on your review of Mountain View Clinic's Policy Manual, do you believe the Policy Manual will assist in protecting the health insurance professional from lawsuit or violations of health care laws and regulations? Explain.

12. We are aware that physicians have a responsibility for their own actions, but what about health insurance professionals? Can the health insurance professional be a party to legal action in the event of error or omission?

 • Keep the Policy Manual open and continue to the next exercise.

Exercise 3

 Online Activity—Identifying Potential Liability, Ethical Issues, and Possible Solutions

 20 minutes

The health insurance professional will have both direct and indirect contact with patients, physicians, clinical staff members, business staff members, and insurance carriers. No matter what position an employee holds or how much education he or she has had, direct and indirect patient contact involves ethical and legal responsibility. The health insurance professional is expected to follow the codes of conduct in health care referred to as medical ethics and medical etiquette.

- Click on the arrow next to **Policy Manual** to expand the menu.
- Click on the arrow next to **Administrative Policies** and then on **Emergency Office Guidelines**. Read from pages 17 through 19 of the Policy Manual.
- Click on **Close Manual** to return to the Reception area.
- Under the Watch heading, click on **Patient Check-In** and watch the video.

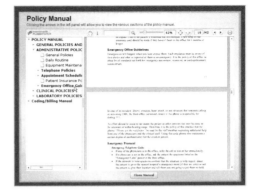

1. Regardless of the health insurance professional's job description or what area of the clinic he or she works from, the health insurance professional must be aware of how to respond to all types of ethical situations that may occur at any location in the office. As you watched the video, what did you observe about Mr. Metcalf's condition?

2. Based on your observations, if you had been assisting Mr. Metcalf, would you have kept him at the counter as Kristin did while she completed the check-in process? Explain your answer.

3. Did Kristin leave herself and the practice open to any potential liability issue(s) in this scene? If so, describe the issue(s) you identified.

4. If Mr. Metcalf had been injured as a result of his fall and the subsequent treatment by the office staff and he chose to pursue legal action against the practice, who would be at risk for liability?
   a. The physicians, the practice, and all three medical assistants
   b. The practice, Charlie, and Kristin
   c. Only Charlie and Kristin
   d. Only Kristin

- Click the **X** on the video screen to close the video.
- Remain in the Reception area with Wilson Metcalf as your patient and continue to the next exercise.

Exercise 4

Online Activity—Breaches of Medical Ethics and Medical Etiquette

20 minutes

- Click on **Policy** to open the office Policy Manual.
- Type "ethics" in the search bar and click once on the magnifying glass.
- Read the section in the Policy Manual concerning "Work Ethics and Professional Behavior."
- Keep the Policy Manual open to answer the following questions.

1. The "Work Ethics and Professional Behavior" section in the Policy Manual notes that employees are to show compassion and care toward patients. Based on these guidelines, describe how Kristin's interaction with Mr. Metcalf in the Patient Check-In video fell short of those guidelines. (*Note:* If necessary, click **Close Manual** to return to Reception and review the Patient Check-In video again.)

Questions 2 through 7 identify some of the medical ethics and etiquette problems that occurred during Wilson Metcalf's Patient Check-In video. In the space below each statement, describe a more appropriate manner to handle the situation.

2. Kristin does not acknowledge Mr. Metcalf's obvious distress.

3. Kristin has Mr. Metcalf stand longer than necessary.

4. Kristin asks for insurance information before establishing the true nature of Mr. Metcalf's medical condition.

5. Kristin asks Mr. Metcalf to update his insurance information instead of first addressing his discomfort.

6. In front of Mr. Metcalf and other patients, Kristin suggests to Charlie that Mr. Metcalf needs soap.

7. Kristin shouts loudly to the other assistants for help and to bring the red folder rather than using the intercom or asking someone personally to get the folder.

8. In addition to Kristin's comments about Mr. Metcalf needing soap, what did you notice about her nonverbal communications throughout the video?

9. Explain why it is important for the health insurance professional, as a team player, to be aware of all situations occurring in the office and to be prepared to address them, regardless of his or her job description.

- Click **Close Manual** to return to the Reception area.
- Click the exit arrow.
- Click **Exit the Program** or, if continuing to a new lesson, click **Return to Map** and then click **Yes** on the pop-up menu.

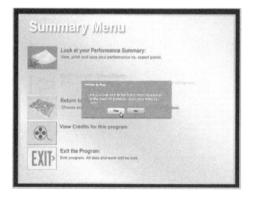

HIPAA Compliance and Privacy in Insurance Billing

Reading Assignment: Chapter 2—HIPAA Compliance and Privacy in Insurance Billing

Patients: Wilson Metcalf, Rhea Davison, Teresa Hernandez, Renee Anderson

Rooms: Exam Room, Reception, Check Out

Objectives:

- Demonstrate an understanding of the Health Insurance Portability and Accountability Act (HIPAA).
- Recognize the organization's Policy Manual as a resource in meeting confidentiality and privacy guidelines.
- Identify the forms used to protect patient privacy.
- Demonstrate the process required for release of information.
- Recognize medical practice confidentiality and privacy issues.
- Identify the elements of a general compliance plan.
- Identify examples of health care fraud.

Exercise 1

 Other Activity—Understanding HIPAA

 10 minutes

1. Match the HIPAA-related terms to the appropriate definition.

HIPAA-Related Term	**Definition**
_____ Compliance	a. A rule, condition, or requirement.
_____ HIPAA Title I	b. The use of discretion in keeping secret information.
_____ HIPAA Title II	c. Aimed at allowing for continuous insurance coverage for workers and their dependents when they change jobs.
_____ Standard	d. Meeting regulations, recommendations, and expectations of federal and state agencies.
_____ Privacy	e. Aimed at reducing health care administrative costs and burdens.
_____ Confidentiality	f. Being secluded from the presence or view of others.

2. Identify the provisions that are included in the Health Insurance Portability and Accountability Act of 1996. Check all that apply.

_____ Lowered administrative costs

_____ Greater access to psychiatric care

_____ Standardized transactions

_____ Limits on the use of preexisting condition exclusions by health insurances

_____ Renewal of health insurance coverage regardless of the individual's health condition

_____ Privacy and security procedures

3. Identify the individuals who can be held accountable for using or disclosing patient health information inappropriately under HIPAA's Privacy Rule. Check all that apply.

_____ Physician

_____ Nurse practitioner

_____ Nurse

_____ Receptionist

_____ Health insurance specialist

_____ Medical transcriptionist

_____ Other patients

Exercise 2

Online Activity—General Confidentiality and Privacy Guidelines

 20 minutes

The health insurance professional has a responsibility to treat all patient information with the highest degree of confidentiality and in accordance with state and federal privacy laws. To ensure compliance with privacy laws, the health insurance professional should be knowledgeable of all federal and state privacy laws. Health insurance professionals should also familiarize themselves with the medical facility's privacy policies.

Note: Keep in mind that privacy policies will vary from practice to practice.

- Sign in to the Mountain View Clinic.
- Select **Wilson Metcalf** from the patient list.
- Click on **Exam Room**.
- Click on **Policy** to open the office Policy Manual.
- Type "HIPAA" in the search bar and click once on the magnifying glass.
- Read the information in the Policy Manual related to HIPAA.
- Click **Close Manual** to return to the Exam Room area.
- Under the Watch heading, click on **Care Coordination** and watch the video.
- Click the **X** on the video screen to close the video.

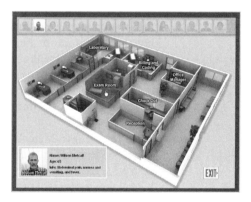

- Click on **Charts**.
- Use Mr. Metcalf's chart and what you observed in the video to answer the following questions.

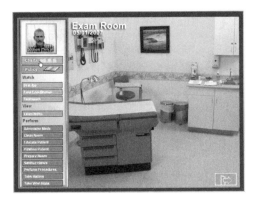

1. According to Mountain View Clinic's Policy Manual, there are six forms that are used with patients in order to implement the HIPAA Privacy Rule. List these six forms.

2. Under what tab in Mr. Metcalf's chart would HIPAA forms allowing release of information for referral purposes be filed?
   a. Patient Information
   b. Patient Medical Information
   c. Hospitalizations
   d. Consultations and Referrals

3. What form was provided to Mr. Metcalf at his initial visit to Mountain View Clinic that informed him of his right to privacy under HIPAA and outlined the complete description of how his health information would be used and/or disclosed?
   a. Notice of Privacy Practices
   b. Acknowledgement of Receipt of Notice of Privacy Practices
   c. Protected Health Information Disclosure Record
   d. Right to Request Confidential Communication Notice

4. What form in Mr. Metcalf's chart was signed by him, ensuring that he has been advised of the office's privacy policies and how his health information will be handled?
   a. Notice of Privacy Practices
   b. Acknowledgement of Receipt of Notice of Privacy Practices
   c. Authorization for Release of Information
   d. Right to Request Confidential Communication Notice

5. What form(s) in Mr. Metcalf's chart are signed and allows the practice to release his information to the hospital?
   a. Acknowledgement of Receipt of Notice of Privacy Practices
   b. Authorization for Release of Information
   c. Protected Health Information Disclosure Record
   d. Request for Correction/Amendment of Protected Health Information

6. On 1/4/2007, Mr. Metcalf agreed to have the practice provide his son Alan with information from the medical record. Of the following, what information was included in this authorization for release?
   a. His entire medical record
   b. All progress notes
   c. Mental health/alcohol and drug abuse treatment
   d. Statement of charges/payments

7. On 1/4/2007, Mr. Metcalf agreed to allow Bristol Medical Center to release information to Dr. Meyer for the purpose of:
   a. continued patient care.
   b. disability determination.
   c. legal purposes.
   d. submission of insurance claims.

8. Under what circumstances would confidentiality between Bristol Medical Center and Mr. Metcalf be automatically waived?
   a. If Bristol Medical Center provided information to the third-party insurance carrier paying Mr. Metcalf's bill
   b. If the state requested Mr. Metcalf's records related to an investigation in which it was suspected that Mr. Metcalf was a victim of elder abuse
   c. If Mr. Metcalf was a member of a managed care organization that requested access to Mr. Metcalf's records for auditing purposes
   d. All of the above
   e. None of the above

- Click **Close Chart** to return to the Exam Room.
- Click the exit arrow.
- Click **Return to Map** and select **Yes** at the pop-up menu to return to the office map.

Exercise 3

Online Activity—Protecting Confidential Information

30 minutes

- Select **Rhea Davison** from the patient list.
- Click on **Reception**.
- Under the Watch heading, click on **Patient Check-In** and watch the video.

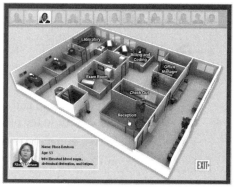

1. Kristin explained to Ms. Davison that she could not provide her with information about her friend Jay because:
   a. Ms. Davison asked him but he did not respond.
   b. the office staff is not allowed to share information about any of their patients.
   c. Kristin cannot verify that Ms. Davison and Jay are friends.
   d. Kristin is not certified.

2. Kristin acknowledges to Ms. Davison that Jay has been in the office a lot lately. This is:
   a. acceptable because she did not explain why he was in the office so much.
   b. acceptable because Ms. Davison was concerned and had no bad intentions.
   c. unacceptable because she should not share any information at all about the patient.
   d. unacceptable because the office manager overheard the conversation.

3. Did the office manager explain the practice's privacy policy well to Ms. Davison? Explain.

4. Did the office manager offer good advice to Kristin and the other staff member regarding privacy issues? Explain.

5. Did Ms. Davison become offended when Kristin explained that she could not share information about her friend Jay? Explain.

- Click the **X** on the video screen to close the video.
- Click the exit arrow.
- Click **Return to Map** and select **Yes** at the pop-up menu to return to the office map.
- Select **Teresa Hernandez** from the patient list.
- Click on **Reception**.
- Under the Watch heading, click on **Patient Check-In** and watch the video.
- Click the **X** on the video screen to close the video.
- Click the exit arrow.
- Click **Return to Map** and select **Yes** at the pop-up menu to return to the office map.
- Click on **Check Out**.

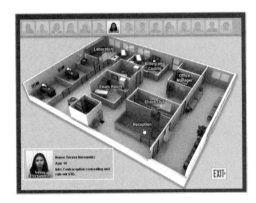

- Under the Watch heading, click on **Patient Check-Out** and watch the video.
- Click the **X** on the video screen to close the video.
- Click on **Charts**.

Teresa Hernandez is a minor seeking contraceptive counseling and STD testing from her physician at Mountain View Clinic on 5/1/2007. She does not want her parents to know that she has come for these services. Answer the following questions to confirm the effectiveness of the actions taken by the staff in protecting the privacy of the patient's visit.

6. Indicate whether each of the following statements is true or false.

    a. _____ The receptionist at Mountain View Clinic provided the patient with an explanation of her privacy rights, and the patient was confident that her health information would be protected as she requested.

    b. _____ The patient was given a Notice of Privacy Practices stating how her health information would be used.

    c. _____ Upon notification by the patient that she did not want her father to receive any information regarding this visit, the receptionist provided the patient with an opportunity to state her request in writing and it was filed in the patient's chart.

    d. _____ Because of the confidential nature of the patient's conversation with the receptionist, care was taken to ensure that other patients in the waiting room were not within hearing range of the conversation.

    e. _____ The physician made a notation on the patient's Encounter Form to remind the health insurance specialist that special privacy precautions should be taken in submitting the claim to the insurance carrier to prevent the parents from receiving information.

    f. _____ Upon check-out, the patient was advised that although the practice would not release any confidential information to the parents, the insurance carrier would send the parents an explanation of benefits and suggested that the patient provide an alternative address where the EOB could be sent.

    g. _____ The alternative address that the patient requested be used to protect her privacy was documented in the chart.

7. Based on this exercise, are you confident that Teresa Hernandez's father will not receive any information regarding her visit to Mountain View Clinic and that the staff has taken all necessary precautions to protect her health information? Discuss steps that could be taken to ensure appropriate precautions have been taken.

8. Identify any reasonable and appropriate safeguards the health insurance specialist can take to ensure that all confidential health information is protected from unauthorized and inappropriate access. Check all that apply.

_____ Do not speak with other staff members during work hours.

_____ Use privacy glass when working in the front desk area.

_____ Do not include PHI on insurance claim forms.

_____ Never use e-mail to transfer PHI.

_____ Keep your computer screen turned so viewing is restricted to authorized staff members only.

_____ Share your password with co-workers only.

_____ Do not place notes with confidential information in areas that are easy to view by nighttime cleaning staff.

_____ Place medical record charts face down on your desk when you are not using them.

_____ Check patient's medical record in the computer system to determine whether there are any special instructions for contacting the patient.

_____ Set your computer to log off automatically after being idle for a period of time.

9. Identify any additional reasonable and appropriate safeguards that the health insurance specialist can take to ensure that confidential health information is protected.

 • Click **Close Chart** to return to the Exam Room.
- Click the exit arrow.
- Click **Return to Map** and select **Yes** at the pop-up menu to return to the office map.
- Select **Renee Anderson** from the patient list.
- Click on **Reception**.
- Under the Watch heading, click on **Patient Check-In** and watch the video.

10. What was Ms. Anderson's concern about her medical records?

11. How did Kristen address this issue?

12. Renee Anderson has a PPO insurance plan under her husband's name. Could this affect the situation in any way? If so, how should the matter be addressed?

 • Click the **X** on the video screen to close the video.
• Remain in the Reception area with Renee Anderson as your patient and continue to the next exercise.

Exercise 4

 Online Activity—Developing a Compliance Plan

 20 minutes

• Click on **Policy** to open the office Policy Manual.
• It is important to be very familiar with your practice's compliance plan. Review Mountain View Clinic's Policy Manual to locate any HIPAA or general compliance information that you can reference.

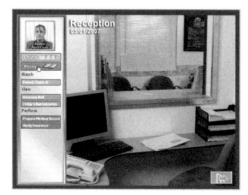

Health care organizations must implement written policies and procedures that comply with HIPAA standards. They should have a policy and procedure manual to train staff and to serve as a resource for situations that need clarification. It is essential that the insurance billing specialist be familiar with the organization's policy and procedure manual and to ask questions about the many aspects of HIPAA or the general operations of the health care organization.

1. Does the office Policy Manual include information regarding HIPAA?
   a. Yes
   b. No

2. What section of the office Policy Manual includes information regarding general compliance of the office?
   a. Work ethics
   b. Telephone policies
   c. Patient insurance policies
   d. Financial policies
   e. Health care fraud and abuse laws
   f. Medical record retention

3. Match each general compliance term with its definition.

General Compliance Term	Definition
_____ Fraud	a. Investigates criminal issues referred by other governing bodies.
_____ Abuse	b. Occurs when deception is used to obtain payment of a claim.
_____ Qui Tam	c. Allows a private citizen to report actions of fraud to the federal government.
_____ CMP	d. Practices that are inconsistent with accepted business standards.
_____ OIG	e. Provides administrative mediation to combat health care fraud and abuse.

4. From your textbook, list the seven basic components of a compliance plan and comment as to whether or not these components are addressed in the office's Policy Manual.

• In a previous exercise, you watched the Check Out video for Teresa Hernandez. The following questions are based on that video. To review the video, click the exit arrow, click **Return to Map** and select **Yes**, select **Teresa Hernandez** and **Check Out**, and click on **Patient Check-Out** to watch the video.

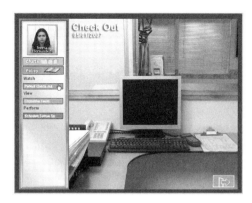

5. Based on Teresa Hernandez's Check-Out video, indicate whether each of the following statements is true or false.

   a. _____ If the office staff offered to waive the $10 copay due by Teresa Hernandez, it could be perceived as an act of health care fraud.

   b. _____ Offering to send correspondence to Teresa Hernandez's boyfriend as an alternative address could be perceived as an act of health care fraud.

   c. _____ The office staff changes the diagnosis on Teresa Hernandez's claim form to "cough" rather than for "contraceptive counseling" so that her father will not know why she was there. This could be perceived as an act of health care fraud.

   d. _____ The office staff contacts Teresa Hernandez's insurance company to request that communications be sent to an alternate address. This could be perceived as an act of health care fraud.

   e. _____ The office staff offers to bill the insurance company under another patient's name so that Teresa Hernandez father will not know why she was at the practice. This could be perceived as an act of health care fraud.

• Click the **X** on the video screen to close the video or click **Close Manual**.
• Click the exit arrow.
• Click **Exit the Program** or, if continuing to a new lesson, click **Return to Map** and then click **Yes** on the pop-up menu.

LESSON 3

Basics of Health Insurance

 Reading Assignment: Chapter 3—Basics of Health Insurance

Patients: All

Rooms: Bill and Coding, Reception, Check Out

Objectives:

- Understand the concepts related to insurance-physician-patient contracts.
- Identify Mountain View Clinic's billing and collection policies related to participating and nonparticipating insurance carriers.
- Determine appropriate actions that the health insurance professional can take to help patients avoid costly outcomes as they deal with insurance policies.
- Identify the sources of health insurance used by Mountain View Clinic patients.
- Determine which, if any, of Mountain View Clinic patients are affected by coordination of benefits, or the "birthday rule."
- Demonstrate the ability to post professional services, fees, payments, adjustments, and balances due to financial accounting records.

Exercise 1

 Online Activity—Contracts in Health Care

20 minutes

- Sign in to Mountain View Clinic.
- Select **John R. Simmons** from the patient list.
- Click on **Billing and Coding**.
- Click on **Charts**.
- Click on the **Patient Information** tab and select **5-Insurance Cards**.

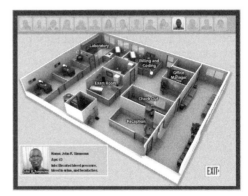

1. Does Dr. Simmons have a contract with an insurance carrier?

2. How would you determine whether a contract between Dr. Simmons and his insurance is implied or expressed?

3. Refer to your textbook to determine the four considerations that were involved when the insurance contract between Dr. Simmons and his insurance carrier was drawn up. List these below.

4. What is the health care provider's promise to Dr. Simmons through their contractual agreement?

5. What is Dr. Simmons' promise to the health care provider through their contract?

6. How would you determine whether the contract between Dr. Simmons and Mountain View Clinic is implied or expressed?

 • Select **Close Chart** to return to the Billing and Coding area.
• Click the exit arrow.
• Click **Return to Map** and select **Yes** at the pop-up menu to return to the office map.

Exercise 2

 Online Activity—Participating Versus Nonparticipating Providers

 30 minutes

• Click on **Reception**.
• Click on **Policy** to open the office Policy Manual.
• Type "Financial Policy" in the search bar and click once on the magnifying glass.
• Read the "Financial Policy" and "Accepted Insurance Carriers and Managed Care Plans" sections that begin on page 32.

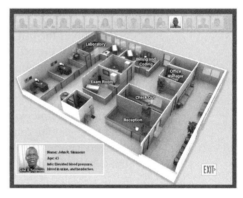

1. According to Mountain View Clinic's Policy Manual, when should the patient be told whether the provider participates with the patient's insurance carrier?
   a. Before the patient schedules the appointment
   b. When the patient checks in for his or her appointment
   c. When the patient checks out from his or her appointment.
   d. When a statement is sent to the patient for payment of the services provided.

2. If the physician at Mountain View Clinic does not participate with the patient's insurance plan, the patient should be informed that the office does not accept the insurance and:
   a. the patient should leave and find services elsewhere.
   b. the patient may schedule an appointment, but payment is expected at the time of service.
   c. the patient may schedule an appointment, and the patient will be billed within 30 days from the date of service.
   d. the patient should be advised to drop the current insurance and find a carrier that the provider participates with.

3. Which of the following health insurance plans does Mountain View Clinic not participate with? Select all that apply.

_____ Blue Cross/Blue Shield

_____ Medicare

_____ Liberty Bell Mutual

_____ Teacher's Health Group

_____ Acme Auto

_____ Workers' Compensation

_____ Small Business Owners' Health

_____ Metropolitan Assurance

_____ Unity Health Care

4. You have just been hired as a health insurance professional at Mountain View Clinic. A staff member at the clinic tells you that insurance cards should be photocopied if the patient's insurance has changed or if the patient has not been in the office for 6 months or longer. You know that this is:
   a. correct only if the office accepts the insurance.
   b. correct even if the office does not accept the insurance.
   c. never correct; it is unnecessary as long as you have updated the information on the Patient Information Form.

5. Mountain View Clinic will file insurance claims with:
   a. indemnity insurance carriers.
   b. managed care plans listed in the Policy Manual.
   c. both a and b.

→ • Click **Close Manual** to return to the Reception area.
• Click the exit arrow.
• Click **Return to Map** and select **Yes** at the pop-up menu to return to the office map.
• Select **Shaunti Begay** from the patient list.
• Click on **Reception**.
• Under the Watch heading, click on **Patient Check-In** and watch the video.
• Click the **X** on the video screen to close the video.
• Click the exit arrow.
• Click **Return to Map** and select **Yes** at the pop-up menu to return to the office map.

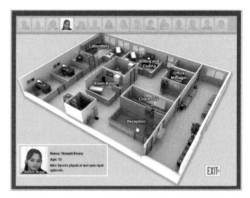

- Click on **Check Out**.
- Under the Watch heading, click on **Patient Check-Out** and watch the video.
- Click the **X** on the video screen to close the video.
- Click on the **Encounter Form** clipboard on the desk.

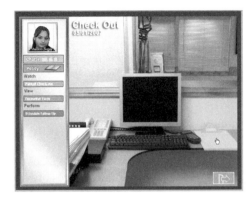

6. How could the problem in the video regarding the patient's insurance have plan been avoided?

7. What information does Kristin give to Shaunti's parents regarding their insurance carrier?

8. What does Kristin offer to do to assist Shaunti's parents with this unfortunate situation? Check all that apply.

_____   Offers to help the family find a participating provider

_____   Offers to help them schedule an appointment with a participating provider

_____   Offers to pay for the visit herself

_____   Offers to let Shaunti keep the appointment with Dr. Haler and warns they will have to pay in full for the visit

_____   Offers to supply an estimate of charges for the day

_____   Offers to waive the charges since the office made a mistake

_____   Suggests they might be reimbursed by Unity Health Care if they file the claim themselves

9. Where would Kristin find the phone number to contact the insurance plan?

10. In the Check-Out video, the Mountain View Clinic staff member had to determine the total fees for the services provided to Shaunti. Where would she locate this information? How much was she required to ask Mr. Begay to pay?

 • Click **Finish** to return to the Check Out area.
 • Click the exit arrow.
 • Click **Return to Map** and select **Yes** at the pop-up menu to return to the office map.

Exercise 3

 Online Activity—Protecting Confidential Information

 40 minutes

 • In this exercise, you will review the insurance coverage for each patient.
 • Select **Janet Jones** from the patient list.
 • On the office map, click on **Check Out**.
 • Click on **Charts**.
 • Review the insurance section of the Patient Information Form. For most patients you can view patient's insurance card(s) by clicking on the **Patient Information** tab and selecting **Insurance Cards**.
 • To view the next patient's chart you must close the chart, exit to the Office Map, select the next patient, reenter the Check Out area, and click on **Charts**. Follow this sequence for each patient as you complete question 1.

1. For each patient listed in the left column on the next two pages:
   • Enter the name of the patient's primary insurer and secondary insurer, if any (in columns 2 and 3).
   • In column 4, write "yes" or "no" to indicate whether or not the clinic will file the patient's insurance claim(s).
   • If the patient has two insurance carriers, provide in column 5 an explanation for sequencing of primary and secondary coverage based on your knowledge of the birthday rule, the definition of supplemental insurance, and the meaning of the birthday rule.

Patient Name	Primary Insurance	Secondary Insurance	Will Clinic File Claim?	Explanation for Coordination of Benefits
Janet Jones				
Wilson Metcalf				
Rhea Davison				
Shaunti Begay				
Jean Deere				
Renee Anderson				
Theresa Hernandez				
Louise Parlet				

Patient Name	Primary Insurance	Secondary Insurance	Will Clinic File Claim?	Explanation for Coordination of Benefits
Tristan Tsosie				
Jose Imero				
Jade Wong				
John R. Simmons				
Hu Huang				
Kevin McKinzie				
Jesus Santo				

Exercise 4

Online Activity—Posting of Professional Services

15 minutes

Complete the following steps to answer questions 1 through 4.

- Select **Rhea Davison** from the patient list.
- Click on **Billing and Coding**.
- Click on the **Encounter Form** clipboard to determine the services that were provided to the patient on 5/1/07.
- Click on the **Fee Schedule** sheet to determine the fee charged by Mountain View Clinic for the services provided.
- Repeat the above steps for **Jean Deere** and **Shaunti Begay**.

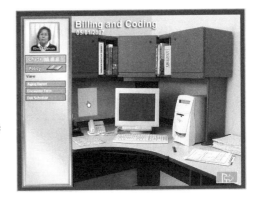

1. Complete the patient ledger for the services provided to **Rhea Davison** on 5/1/07. Also post any previous balances or payment made on that date.

Mountain View Clinic
Patient Ledger

DATE:
Patient ID:
Patient Name:
Insurance Type:

Date	Professional Service	Fee ($)	Payment ($)	Adj. ($)	Prev. Bal. ($)	New Balance ($)
Totals						

2. Complete the patient ledger for the services provided to **Jean Deere** on 5/1/07. Also post any previous balances or payments made on that date.

Mountain View Clinic
Patient Ledger

DATE:

Patient ID:

Patient Name:

Insurance Type:

Date	Professional Service	Fee ($)	Payment ($)	Adj. ($)	Prev. Bal. ($)	New Balance ($)
Totals						

3. Complete the patient ledger for the services provided to **Shaunti Begay** on 5/1/07. Also post any previous balances or payments made on that date.

Mountain View Clinic
Patient Ledger

DATE:
Patient ID:
Patient Name:
Insurance Type:

Date	Professional Service	Fee ($)	Payment ($)	Adj. ($)	Prev. Bal. ($)	New Balance ($)
Totals						

4. Post the transactions for **Rhea Davison**, **Jean Deere**, and **Shaunti Begay** occurring on 5/1/07 to the daysheet provided below.

Mountain View Clinic
Daysheet

Date	Professional Service	Fee	Payment	Adjustment	New Balance	Old Balance	Patient's Name	Distribution	
								Dr. Hayler	Dr. Meyer
TOTALS									**TOTALS**

• Click **Finish** to return to the Billing and Coding area.

• Click the exit arrow.

• Click **Exit the Program** or, if continuing to a new lesson, click **Return to Map** and then click **Yes** on the pop-up menu.

LESSON 4

Medical Documentation

 Reading Assignment: Chapter 4—Medical Documentation and the Electronic Health Record

Patients: Wilson Metcalf, Tristan Tsosie

Rooms: Reception, Exam Room, Billing and Coding

Objectives:

- Recognize the importance of the organization's medical record policies.
- Identify Mountain View Clinic's medical record policies.
- Identify the elements of a medical record and locate them in the chart.
- Correctly update patient information in the medical record.
- Identify specific details of documentation within the medical record to support services billed.
- Identify specific elements of the physician's documentation

Exercise 1

 Online Activity—General Medical Records Guidelines

25 minutes

The medical record serves many purposes in the medical practice. It is the source of information used for the health insurance professional to submit accurate insurance claims. Therefore the health insurance professional must be knowledgeable of all federal, state, and local regulations related to medical records. Keep in mind that policies will vary from practice to practice and from state to state. A critical step in the proper handling of medical records begins with the health insurance professional becoming familiar with the medical facility's medical record policies.

- Sign in to the Mountain View Clinic.
- Select **Wilson Metcalf** from the patient list.
- Click on **Reception**.
- Click on **Policy** to open the office Policy Manual.
- Review all of Mountain View Clinic's policies regarding medical records.

77

Copyright © 2012 by Saunders, an imprint of Elsevier Inc. All rights reserved.

Use the information provided in the Mountain View Clinic's Policy Manual to answer the following questions.

1. According to Mountain View Clinic's Policy Manual, what step should you, as the health insurance professional, take to ensure continuity of patient care when medical records are used?
   a. Tell the receptionist that you have taken the patient's record.
   b. Sign out any patient record you have taken.
   c. Return the chart within 24 hours.
   d. Just use common sense.

2. At Mountain View Clinic, a medical record progress note must be completed by the physician and placed in the chart:
   a. as soon as the patient leaves the office.
   b. as soon as the dictation has been transcribed.
   c. within 24 hours from the date of service.
   d. within 14 days from the date of service.

3. According to Mountain View Clinic's Policy Manual, the health insurance professional should ask for clarification regarding charges and associated documentation submitted by a physician:
   a. within 14 days from the date of service.
   b. after the claim has been billed.
   c. upon the request for clarification from the insurance carrier.
   d. never; there is no need for clarification because reporting of charges and associated documentation is the physician's responsibility.

4. At Mountain View Clinic, any adult's medical record will be maintained:
   a. as long as the adult is a patient at the clinic.
   b. for a period of 3 years from the last date of service.
   c. for a period of 15 years from the last date of service.
   d. for a period of 15 years from the time the adult leaves the practice.

5. After the minimum retention time has been met, outside vendors to Mountain View Clinic should dispose of records by:
   a. returning them to the clinic.
   b. dropping them off at the local recycling center.
   c. putting them in a garbage pick-up area.
   d. shredding or burning them.

6. Why is it important for the health insurance professional to be knowledgeable of all medical record policies ?

 • Click **Close Manual** to return to the Reception area.
• Remain in the Reception area with Wilson Metcalf as your patient to continue to the next exercise.

Exercise 2

 Online Activity—Components of the Medical Record—Patient Information

 25 minutes

It is essential for the health insurance professional to be familiar with all components of the medical record and where they are placed.

 • Click on **Charts** to open Mr. Metcalf's medical record and review all components of the medical record.

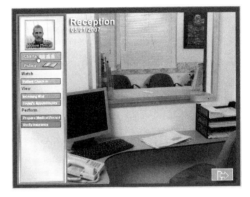

1. Copies of the patient's insurance card(s) are included under which tab?
   a. Patient Information
   b. Patient Medical Information
   c. Hospitalization
   d. Workers' Comp

2. The patient's medication record is included under which tab?
   a. Patient Information
   b. Patient Medical Information
   c. Diagnostic Tests
   d. Hospitalization

3. There is no information located in Mr. Metcalf's chart under which tab at the present time?
   a. Patient Medical Information
   b. Diagnostic Tests
   c. Hospitalization
   d. Workers' Comp

4. IP Progress Notes are listed twice under the Hospitalization tab because:
   a. the record has been duplicated in error.
   b. another patient's record has been filed in Mr. Metcalf's chart in error.
   c. there are two different dates of service.
   d. there are two different records from two different physicians.

5. Using all information and forms found under the Patient Information tab of Mr. Metcalf's chart, identify whether each of the following statements is true or false.

    a. _____ There are two Patient Information Forms in Wilson Metcalf's chart.

    b. _____ Based on patient registration information available on 1/4/2007, the patient's mailing address is 148 Zenith Blvd., London, XY 55555.

    c. _____ According to the Primary Insurance section of the Patient Information Form dated 1/4/2007, Mr. Metcalf's primary insurance is Independent Contractor's Group.

    d. _____ Mr. Metcalf has one insurance card on file at Mountain View Clinic.

    e. _____ Mr. Metcalf's Medicare insurance card states that his coverage became effective on 4/6/2007.

    f. _____ According to Mr. Metcalf's updated Patient Information Form dated 5/1/2007, his primary insurance is Independent Contractor's Group insurance.

6. Why is it important for the health insurance professional to be able to locate components of the medical record?

 • Click **Close Chart** to return to the Reception area.

• Remain in the Reception area with Wilson Metcalf as your patient and continue to the next exercise.

Exercise 3

 Online Activity—Updating Patient Information in the Medical Record

 20 minutes

• Under the Watch heading, click on **Patient Check-In** and watch the video.

• Pause the video when Mr. Metcalf begins to look for his insurance card (click on the pause button in the lower left hand corner of the video screen).

• Click the **X** on the video screen to close the video.

• Click on **Charts**.

• Click on the **Patient Information** tab and select **2-Insurance Cards**.

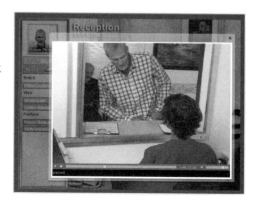

1. Using the new insurance card in Mr. Metcalf's chart, update the Primary Insurance section of his Patient Information Form below.

PRIMARY INSURANCE

Person Responsible for Account _____

Last Name   First Name   Initial

Relation to Patient _____ Birthdate _____ Soc. Sec.# _____

Address (if different from patient's) _____ Phone _____

City _____ State _____ Zip _____

Person Responsible Employed by _____ Occupation _____

Business Address _____ Business Phone _____

Insurance Company _____

Contract # _____ Group # _____ Subscriber # _____

Name of other dependents covered under this plan _____

ADDITIONAL INSURANCE

Is patient covered by additional insurance? ____ Yes ____ No

Subscriber Name _____ Relation to Patient _____ Birthdate _____

Address (if different from patient's) _____ Phone _____

City _____ State _____ Zip _____

Subscriber Employed by _____ Business Phone _____

Insurance Company _____ Soc. Sec.# _____

Contract # _____ Group # _____ Subscriber # _____

Name of other dependents covered under this plan _____

---

2. Kristin, the receptionist, asks Mr. Metcalf whether there has been a change in his insurance. What is his response?

- Click **Close Chart** to return to the Reception area.
- Click the exit arrow.
- Click **Return to Map** and select **Yes** at the pop-up menu to return to the office map.

Exercise 4

 Online Activity—Identifying Components of the Medical Record

 25 minutes

A function of the medical record is to provide support for billing of services and third-party reimbursement. Lack of proper documentation can result in reduced or denied claim payment. Therefore the health insurance professional must be adept at finding specific details of information within the medical record.

- On the office map, click on **Exam Room**.
- Click on **Charts** to open Mr. Metcalf's medical record and review all components of the medical record.
- Click **Close Chart** to return to the Exam Room.
- Click on the **Exam Notes** file folder to read the documentation regarding Mr. Metcalf's visit.

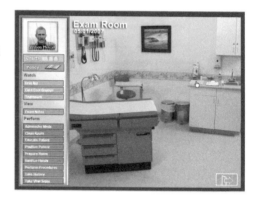

1. On what date was Mr. Metcalf's General Health History taken?

2. According to Mr. Metcalf's General Health History, what was his mother's cause of death?

3. What three medications was Mr. Metcalf taking when he came to the practice on 1/4/2007?

4. Did Mr. Metcalf have any previous diagnostic tests performed? If so, what test(s) and when?

5. According to Mr. Metcalf's records, how many previous visits to the hospital has he had?

6. Why was Mr. Metcalf admitted to the hospital on 4/9/1994?

7. Whose signature appears at the end of the Progress Note dated 5/1/2007?

8. What was the chief complaint documented in Dr. Meyer's Exam Note of 5/1/2007?

9. What is the final diagnosis documented in Dr. Meyer's Exam Note of 5/1/2007?

10. Separate from the medical record, where would an itemization of the services being billed on 5/1/2007 be located?

11. If the health insurance professional determines that the patient did not sign his exam note, why is it important to bring it to Dr. Meyer's attention?

→ • Click **Finish** to return to the Exam Room.
 • Click the exit arrow.
 • Click **Return to Map** and select **Yes** at the pop-up menu to return to the office map.

Exercise 5

Online Activity—Identifying Elements of the Patient Visit

20 minutes

- Select **Tristan Tsosie** from the patient list.
- Click on **Billing and Coding**.
- Click on **Charts**.
- Click on the **Consultation & Referral** tab and select **1-Consultation Notes**.

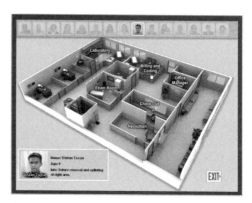

1. What is the patient's chief complaint?

2. Which of the key elements of an evaluation and management note are included as part of this Consultation Note? Check all that apply.

_____ History

_____ Exam

_____ Medical decision making

3. Which elements of the history are documented in the Consultation Note? Check all that apply.

_____ Chief complaint

_____ History of present illness

_____ Review of systems

_____ Past history

_____ Family history

_____ Social history

4. Which elements of HPI are supported in the corresponding documentation? Check all that apply.

_____ Location

_____ Quality

_____ Severity

_____ Duration

_____ Timing

_____ Context

_____ Modifying factors

_____ Associated signs and symptoms

5. Which elements of this note are considered part of the medical decision making process? Check all that apply.

_____ Medications

_____ Physical exam

_____ Imaging

_____ Assessment

_____ Plan

6. Why would it be necessary for the health insurance professional to perform an internal audit of the medical record to ensure that these elements of the patient visit have been adequately documented?

➤ • Click **Close Chart** to return to the Billing and Coding area.
  • Click the exit arrow.
  • Click **Return to Map**, then click **Yes** at the pop-up menu to return to the office map or click **Exit the Program**.

LESSON 5

Diagnostic Coding

 Reading Assignment: Chapter 5—Diagnostic Coding

Patients: Jean Deere, Jose Imero, Kevin McKinzie

Rooms: Exam Room, Billing and Coding

Resources Needed: Current Year ICD-9-CM Coding Manual

Objectives:

- Identify guidelines available in the ICD-9-CM manual to assist in accurate diagnosis coding.
- Demonstrate an understanding of the ICD-9-CM coding process by accurately assigning codes to diagnosis lists.
- Demonstrate an understanding of the ICD-9-CM coding process by accurately coding patients' diagnoses to the greatest degree of specificity.

Exercise 1

 Writing Activity—Identifying the ICD-9-CM Coding Process and Guidelines

25 minutes

To become a proficient coder, it is important to develop an understanding of the conventions, terminology, and guidelines for ICD-9-CM coding, which are included in the ICD-9-CM coding manual. These rules assist in the selection of correct diagnosis codes for the patient's encounter. The insurance billing specialist must be familiar with the location of the guidelines and access them when assigning diagnosis codes. The following is an exercise to assist in identifying the guidelines in the coding manual.

1. Locate the instructional steps for using Physician's Volumes 1 & 2 of the ICD-9-CM manual and outline the essential steps of diagnostic coding by completing the statements below.

   a. Locate the diagnosis in the patient's _____ _____.

   b. Determine the _____ _____ of the stated diagnosis.

   c. Find the main term in the _____ _____ _____.

d. Read and apply any _____ or _____.

e. Cross-reference the code found to the _____ _____

_____.

f. Read and be guided by the _____ and _____.

g. Read through the entire category and code the highest level of _____.

2. Never code directly from the _____ _____.

Locate the Official Coding Guidelines in the ICD-9-CM manual to answer the following questions.

3. The Official Coding Guidelines (Section I.A.9) state that the instruction _____ _____ following a main term in the index instructs that another main term may also be referenced and may provide additional entries that might be useful.

4. The Official Coding Guidelines (Section I.B.3) state that diagnosis codes are to be used at their _____ number of digits available.

5. In the Official Coding Guidelines (Section I.B.6), it states that codes for _____ and _____, as opposed to diagnoses, are acceptable for reporting purposes when a related definitive diagnosis has not been established.

6. As stated in the Official Coding Guidelines (Section I.C.19.a.5), the selection of the appropriate E code is guided by the _____ to _____ _____.

7. As stated in the Official Coding Guidelines (Section 1.C.19.a.6), an E code can never be listed _____ or in the _____ _____.

8. The Official Coding Guidelines (Section I.C.19.a.3) state to use the full range of E codes to completely describe the cause, the intent, and the _____ of _____.

9. As stated in the Official Coding Guidelines (Section IV.I), when coding outpatient services, do not code diagnoses documented as "probable," "suspected," "questionable," or "_____ _____."

10. As stated in the Official Coding Guidelines (Section IV.K), when coding outpatient services, code all documented conditions that coexist at the time of the encounter and require or affect patient care, _____, or _____.

Exercise 2

Online Activity—Applying the ICD-9-CM Coding Process and Guidelines

 15 minutes

- Sign in to the Mountain View Clinic
- Select **Jean Deere** from the patient list.
- Click on **Exam Room**.
- Click on the **Exam Notes** file folder.

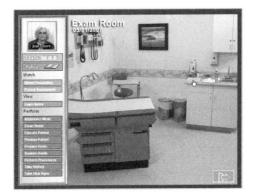

1. Under the Impression portion of the Exam Notes for Jean Deere, the physician states that the patient has a "mild to moderate memory loss." Below, work through the process for selecting the appropriate ICD-9-CM code for this condition.

Main Term	Diagnosis Code Indicated in the Alphabetic Index	Diagnosis Code Confirmed by Tabular List

2. Under the Impression portion of the Exam Notes for Jean Deere, the physician states that the patient has "impaired hearing." Below, work through the process for selecting the appropriate ICD-9-CM code for this condition.

Main Term	Diagnosis Code Indicated in the Alphabetic Index	Diagnosis Code Confirmed by Tabular List

3. Under the Impression portion of the Exam Notes for Jean Deere, the physician states that the patient has "ear pain." Below, work through the process for selecting the appropriate ICD-9-CM code for this condition.

Main Term	Diagnosis Code Indicated in the Alphabetic Index	Diagnosis Code Confirmed by Tabular List

- Click **Finish** to return to the Exam Room.
- Click the exit arrow.
- On the Summary Menu, click **Return to Map** and select **Yes** at the pop-up menu to return to the office map.

Exercise 3

 Writing Activity—Applying Accurate Codes to the Diagnoses Listed on the Encounter Form

 70 minutes

1. The staff members at Mountain View Clinic have decided to update their Encounter Form with the diagnoses most frequently reported by their practice. Using the most recent edition of the ICD-9-CM codebook and the coding steps presented in the textbook, insert the correct diagnosis codes for each of the given conditions listed on the form below.

_____ Abscess	_____ Bursitis	_____ Fracture	_____ Pneumonia
_____ Abrasion-Sup.Injury	_____ CAD	_____ Gastritis	_____ Pregnancy
_____ Acne	_____ Chest Pain	_____ Gastroenteritis	_____ Rectal Bleed
_____ Alcohol Abuse	_____ CHF	_____ Gout	_____ Sinusitis
_____ Allergic Reaction	_____ Conjunctivitis	_____ Headache	_____ STD _____
_____ Amenorrhea	_____ COPD	_____ Hematuria	_____ Tendonitis
_____ Anemia	_____ Contraception	_____ Hemorrhoids	_____ UTI
_____ Anxiety	_____ Cough	_____ HIV	_____ URI
_____ Annual GYN exam	_____ CVA	_____ Hypertension	_____ Vaginitis
_____ Annual PE	_____ Depression	_____ Hypothyroidism	_____ Well Baby/Child
_____ Arrhythmia	_____ Dermatitis	_____ IBS	_____ Weight Loss
_____ Arthritis	_____ Diabetes*	_____ Low Back Pain	_____ Otitis Media
_____ ASHD	_____ Diarrhea	_____ Lymphadenopathy	_____
_____ Asthma	_____ Dysmenorrheal	_____ Nausea/Vomiting	_____
_____ Backache	_____ Ear Impaction	_____ Obesity	_____
_____ Breast Mass	_____ Fatigue	_____ Osteoporosis	_____
_____ Bronchitis	_____ Fever	_____ Pharyngitis	_____

Exercise 4

 Online Activity—Diagnostic Coding for Jose Imero

 15 minutes

- Select **Jose Imero** from the patient list.
- Click on **Exam Room**.
- Click on the **Exam Notes** file folder.

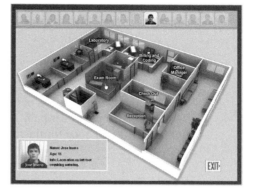

1. Based on the Exam Notes, identify why the patient is being seen today.

2. Below, work through the process for selecting the appropriate diagnosis code for the condition identified in question 1.

Main Term	Diagnosis Code Indicated in the Alphabetic Index	Diagnosis Code Confirmed by Tabular List

3. When you located the main term in the ICD-9-CM, what instructional note did you have to follow?

 4. In addition to reporting the appropriate diagnosis code for this condition, the health insurance specialist is required to report an E code. Review the Official Coding Guidelines from the ICD-9-CM manual and using the E code index, record the appropriate code below to describe how the injury occurred.

Main Term	Diagnosis Code Indicated in the Alphabetic Index	Diagnosis Code Confirmed by Tabular List

5. The Official Coding Guidelines state that the place of occurrence should also be recorded (if it is identified) by reporting an additional E code. Using the E code Index, identify the appropriate code below to describe where the injury occurred.

Main Term	Diagnosis Code Indicated in the Alphabetic Index	Diagnosis Code Confirmed by Tabular List

- Click **Finish** to return to the Exam Room.
- Click the exit arrow.
- Click **Return to Map** and select **Yes** at the pop-up menu to return to the office map.

Exercise 5

Online Activity—Diagnostic Coding for Kevin McKinzie

30 minutes

- Select **Kevin McKinzie** from the patient list.
- Click on **Exam Room**.
- Under the Watch heading, click on **Patient Interview** and watch the video.

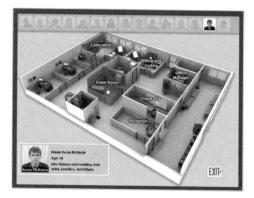

1. During the patient interview, what symptoms does the patient claim to have?

- Click the **X** on the video screen to close the video.
- Click on the **Exam Notes** file folder.

2. In the second sentence of the Exam Notes for this patient, what symptoms does the physician document as the reason for the patient's visit today?

3. In the Exam Notes for this patient, what health problems does the physician document under Impression?

4. One entry in the Impression portion of the Exam Notes is worded "R/O hepatitis, mono." What is the rule about coding an entry like this?

5. When should an ICD-9-CM code be assigned to impressions documented as symptoms or worded as "rule out"?

 • Click **Finish** to return to the Exam Room.
- Click the exit arrow.
- Click **Return to Map** and select **Yes** at the pop-up menu to return to the office map.
- Click on **Billing and Coding**.
- Click on the **Encounter Form** clipboard.

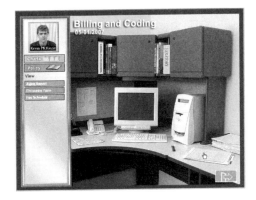

6. Indicate whether each of the following statements is true or false.

a. _____ The diagnoses indicated on Kevin McKinzie's Encounter Form are the same as those documented under Impression in the Exam Notes.

b. _____ In Block 21 of the CMS-1500, the biller/coder should report the conditions/ diagnoses documented in the patient's medical chart, as opposed to those noted on the Encounter Form.

7. When the diagnoses listed on the Encounter Form are different from those documented in the medical record, the biller/coder should:
   a. report only the diagnosis codes noted on the Encounter Form.
   b. report only the diagnosis codes documented in the medical record.
   c. report both the diagnosis codes documented in the record and on the Encounter Form.
   d. report the discrepancy to the physician and ask for clarification regarding what specific diagnoses to code and report.
   e. insert an "addendum" to the medical record, adding the missing diagnoses codes from the Encounter Form.

8. Based on the supporting documentation, indicate which conditions should be reported on Kevin McKinzie's CMS-1500 claim form. Select all that apply.

_____ Dark urine

_____ Low-grade fever

_____ Asthma, well controlled

_____ Nausea w/vomiting

_____ Severe fatigue

_____ Weight loss

_____ Stomach pains

_____ GI symptoms

_____ Jaundice

_____ Yellow eyes

_____ R/O hepatitis/mono

_____ Seizure disorder

9. Of the conditions you did not select in question 8, choose four of these and explain below why these conditions would not be reported.

10. Indicate the appropriate ICD-9-CM code for each condition listed below.

Condition	ICD-9 Code
Asthma, well controlled	
Dark urine	
Fatigue	
Jaundice	
Low-grade fever	
Nausea/vomiting	
Seizure disorder	
Stomach pains	
Weight loss	

- Click **Finish** to return to the Billing and Coding area.
- Click on the exit arrow.
- Click **Exit the Program** or, if continuing to a new lesson, click **Return to Map** and then click **Yes** on the pop-up menu.

LESSON 6

Procedural Coding (E&M and HCPCS)

Reading Assignment: Chapter 6—Procedural Coding

Patients: Jean Deere, Wilson Metcalf, Teresa Hernandez

Room: Billing and Coding

Resources Needed: Current-Year CPT-4 Manual

Objectives:

- Identify guidelines available in the CPT-4 manual to assist in accurate procedural coding.
- Demonstrate an understanding of the CPT coding process by accurately assigning codes to procedural lists.
- Assign correct CPT codes to services/procedures provided to selected patients.
- Demonstrate usage of modifiers when appropriate.

Exercise 1

Writing Activity—Identifying the CPT Coding Process and Guidelines

15 minutes

Before attempting to code a procedure, the health insurance professional must become familiar with the contents and structure of the CPT-4 manual and the process for selecting the appropriate code. Guidelines are included throughout the CPT-4 manual to further assist the health insurance professional in accurately reporting procedure codes. These guidelines should be referenced at all times.

1. Using your textbook, locate the essential steps of procedural coding and identify them by completing the statements below and on the next page.

   a. Identify the _____, _____, or

   _____ to be coded.

97

b. Look up the main term identified in the _____ _____ of the CPT-4 manual.

c. Cross-reference the CPT code(s) located in the index in the _____

_____ of the CPT-4 manual.

d. Read and follow any notes, special instructions, or _____ associated with the code.

e. Determine and _____ the appropriate code.

Using the Introduction of your CPT-4 manual, locate the guidelines that will assist you in accurate procedural coding. Use this information to complete the following statements.

2. Any service or procedure reported with a CPT code must be adequately

_____ in the medical record.

3. If no specific CPT code exists that identifies the services performed, then report the service

using the appropriate _____ procedure code.

4. Instructions, typically included as _____ notes with selected codes, indicate that a code should not be reported with another code or codes.

5. _____ _____ are always performed in addition to the primary service or procedure and must never be reported as stand-alone codes.

6. A _____ provides the means to report or indicate that a performed service or procedure has been altered by some specific circumstance but has not changed in its definition or code.

7. A service that is rarely provided, unusual, variable, or new may require a

_____ _____.

8. The CPT-4 manual features an expandable alphabetical index that includes listings by

_____ and _____ _____.

Exercise 2

Writing Activity—Basic CPT Code Assignment

40 minutes

Mountain View Clinic needs your help! The AMA has just released the new CPT codes for the year, and the coder needs to ensure that the correct codes are on the office Encounter Form. Using your CPT-4 manual, identify the appropriate codes for each procedure listed on the Encounter Form.

1. Using your CPT-4 manual, identify the appropriate codes for each type of office visit listed on the Encounter Form.

New and Established Office Visits	CPT Code
New patient office visit: Level 1	
New patient office visit: Level 2	
New patient office visit: Level 3	
New patient office visit: Level 4	
New patient office visit: Level 5	
Established office visit: Level 1	
Established office visit: Level 2	
Established office visit: Level 3	
Established office visit: Level 4	
Established office visit: Level 5	

2. Using your CPT-4 manual, identify the appropriate codes for each preventive visit listed on the Encounter Form.

New and Established Preventive Care	CPT Code
New preventive care: <1 year	
New preventive care: 1-4 years	
New preventive care: 5-11 years	
New preventive care: 12-17 years	
New preventive care: 18-39 years	
New preventive care: 40-64 years	
New preventive care: 65+ years	

New and Established Preventive Care	CPT Code
Established preventive care: <1 years	
Established preventive care: 1-4 years	
Established preventive care: 5-11 years	
Established preventive care: 12-17 years	
Established preventive care: 18-39 years	
Established preventive care: 40-64 years	
Established preventive care: 65+ years	

 3. Using your CPT-4 manual, identify the appropriate codes for each hospital visit listed on the Encounter Form.

Hospital Visits	CPT Code
Initial hospital care/Admit (low)	
Initial hospital care/Admit (moderate)	
Initial hospital care/Admit (high)	
Subsequent hospital care (low)	
Subsequent hospital care (moderate)	
Subsequent hospital care (high)	
Hospital discharge (30 minutes or less)	
Hospital discharge (more than 30 minutes)	

 4. Using your CPT-4 manual, identify the appropriate codes for each procedure listed on the Encounter Form.

Procedure	CPT Code
Anoscopy; diagnostic	
Audiometry; pure tone (air only)	
Avulsion of nail plate; single	
Burn treatment; initial (local)	
Crutches	
I&D abscess; simple	

Procedure	CPT Code
EKG; tracing, interpretation, and report	
Ear lavage/cerumen removal	
Nebulizer treatment	
Pulse oximetry	
Repair; simple	
Repair; intermediate	
Repair; complex	
Splint; short arm (static)	
Spirometry	
Surgical tray	
Visual acuity screening	

 5. Using your CPT-4 manual, identify the appropriate codes for each immunization listed on the Encounter Form.

Immunization	CPT Code
DT; less than 7 years old; IM	
DTAP; less than 7 years old; IM	
DTP; IM	
Hep B; adult; IM	
Hep B; ped/adolescent; IM	
HIB; IM (3 dose schedule)	
Influenza; IM, 3 years and older	
IPV; polio; IM or subcutaneous	
MMR; subcutaneous	
OPV	
Pneumococcal vaccine; IM or subcutaneous	
Skin Test; TB, intradermal	
TB Tine	
Tetanus; IM	

6. Using your CPT-4 manual, identify the appropriate codes for each injection administration code listed on the Encounter Form.

Injection Administration	CPT Code
Antibiotic; IM	
Immunization; single (no counseling provided)	
Immunization; each additional (no counseling provided)	
Therapeutic injection; IM	
Specific drug	

 7. Using your CPT-4 manual, identify the appropriate codes for each laboratory service listed on the Encounter Form.

Laboratory	CPT Code
Blood sugar; reagent strip	
CBC; automated	
DNA probe	
Epstein-Barr virus screen/Mono screening (Heterophile antibodies screening)	
Handling/Collection	
Hemoccult (blood occult by peroxidase activity)	
Hemoglobin	
KOH slide (tissue examination for fungi, ectoparasite ova or mites)	
Pap smear, slides; manual screening under physician supervision	
Rapid Strep (Streptococcus, Group A)	
UA, dipstick; non-automated with microscopy	
Urine pregnancy test	
Venipuncture	
Wet mount (smear)	

Exercise 3

Online Activity—CPT Coding Assignment 1

30 minutes

- Sign in to the Mountain View Clinic.
- Select **Jean Deere** from the patient list.
- Click on **Billing and Coding**.
- Click on the **Encounter Form** clipboard.

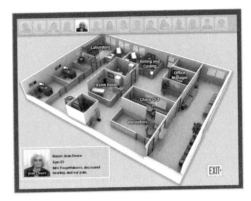

1. Ms. Deere is an established patient, and her office visit is a level IV visit. What is the correct E&M code for this visit level?

2. The procedures/services provided to Ms. Deere today include (1) ear lavage; (2) UA, dipstick; and (3) pulse oximetry. Using the most recent CPT-4 coding manual, provide the correct CPT codes for these three services/procedures.

3. To report the office visit and the surgical procedure provided to Ms. Deere on the same date of service, would it be necessary to report a modifier? If so, what is the purpose of a modifier and which modifier would be most appropriate?

4. Suppose Dr. Meyers admits Ms. Deere to the hospital. What is the E&M code for Dr. Meyer's admission and initial hospital care requiring a moderate complexity of medical decision making?

5. If Dr. Meyers admitted Ms. Deere to the hospital on the same date that he saw her in the office, which E&M service would he report?

6. What code would be used for Dr. Meyers' subsequent hospital visits (moderate complexity) to Ms. Deere?

7. How many of the key components (history, examination, and medical decision making) must the physician meet or exceed in his documentation to support the code you identified in question 6?

8. Assume that during Ms. Deere's hospital stay, tests indicate a heart problem, prompting Dr. Meyers to call in a cardiologist, Dr. Hudson. Dr. Hudson's inpatient consultation includes a comprehensive history, a comprehensive evaluation, and medical decision making of moderate complexity. What is the correct E&M code for Dr. Hudson's consultation?

9. If the consulting physician, Dr. Hudson, sees Ms. Deere a second time during her inpatient stay, what range of CPT codes would Dr. Hudson report?

10. Dr. Meyers spends 20 minutes with Ms. Deere on the last day of her hospitalization, which includes her discharge. The correct code would be _____.

11. If Ms. Deere had been admitted and discharged on the same date by Dr. Meyers, what range of CPT codes would be reported by the physician?

• Click **Finish** to return to the Billing and Coding area.
 • Click the exit arrow.
 • Click **Return to Map** and select **Yes** at the pop-up menu to return to the office map.

Exercise 4

 ### Online Activity—CPT Coding Assignment 2

 20 minutes

 • Select **Wilson Metcalf** from the patient list.
 • Click on **Billing and Coding**.
 • Click on **Charts**.
 • Click on the **Patient Medical Information** tab and select **1-Progress Notes**.

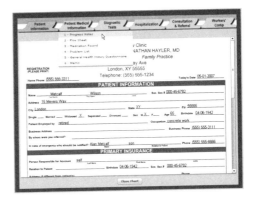

1. Were any laboratory tests completed for Mr. Metcalf on 5/1/2007? If so, list and code each test.

2. Besides the examination, were any procedures performed on 5/1/2007? If so, list and code each.

 3. We know that Mr. Metcalf was subsequently admitted to the hospital. Let's look at a hypothetical scenario for his hospital stay. Assume that he had the following procedures performed in an attempt to acquire a definitive diagnosis: (1) flexible esophagoscopy (2) flexible colonoscopy, proximal to splenic flexure, with removal of two polyps; and (3) needle biopsy of the liver. From blood tests performed by the ED physician, it was determined that Mr. Metcalf was severely anemic. As a result, he was given a blood transfusion. Using the most recent CPT-4 manual, code these four procedures.

4. The use of modifiers in CPT coding can indicate that a service or procedure has been altered by some specific circumstance, but without changing its definition or code. Let's assume that documentation states that the liver biopsy took considerably more time than is typically required. Identify which modifier would be used in this example.

5. The physician's documentation states that approximately halfway through Mr. Metcalf's colonoscopy, the procedure was terminated because his blood pressure dropped and it would have been dangerous to complete the procedure. What modifier would be appended to the colonoscopy to explain that the procedure was not completed?

6. According to Mr. Metcalf's medical record, the flexible esophagoscopy and flexible colonoscopy were performed on the same date of service. What modifier would need to be appended to the second procedure reported on the CMS-1500 claim form?

7. On the last day of his hospitalization, Mr. Metcalf underwent a needle biopsy of the prostate. The correct CPT code for this procedure is _____.

8. If it was documented that ultrasonic imaging guidance was used to perform the needle biopsy of the prostate described above, the CPT code reported for this procedure would be _____.

9. As Mr. Metcalf's needle biopsy was performed, a self-employed radiologist hired by the hospital interpreted the procedure and dictated a radiology report. He will be billing for the professional component of the procedure reported in question 8. What modifier will the radiologist append to the procedure code? What modifier will the hospital append to the procedure code?

10. Wilson Metcalf was discharged from the hospital on day 4. The physician documents that he spent a total of 45 minutes documenting the medical record and then discussing test results, prognoses, and medication requirements with the patient and his son. The correct CPT code for hospital discharge is _____.

11. On the date of discharge, the attending physician called in a podiatrist to treat an area of cellulitis on Mr. Metcalf's left foot. What range of codes would the podiatrist use to report these concurrent care services?

- Click **Close Chart** to return to the Billing and Coding area.
- Click the exit arrow.
- Click **Return to Map** and select **Yes** at the pop-up menu to return to the office map.

Exercise 5

Online Activity—CPT Coding Assignment 3

 20 minutes

- Select **Teresa Hernandez** from the patient list.
- Click on **Billing and Coding**.
- Click on **Charts**.
- Click on the **Patient Medical Information** tab and select **1-Progress Notes**.
- Review the Progress Notes for 5/1/2007.
- Click **Close Chart** to return to the Billing and Coding area.
- Click on the **Encounter Form** clipboard.

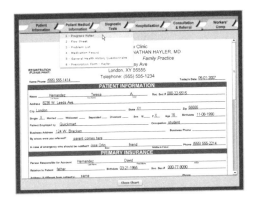

1. List and code all procedures and/or services that were performed on this date.

2. Let's assume that because of Teresa's multiple concurrent problems, her visit (including examination, assessment, and counseling) took much longer than usual. The physician spent a total of 90 minutes face to face with the patient. Is there a method to report this additional time?

3. If it is determined that Teresa has an STD and the physician decides to treat her with an antibiotic injection, what type of code will be used to report the medication being administered?

4. Teresa will return in 3 weeks for a Pap test. The CPT code used for this test will be

   _____.

5. Teresa was given a prescription for a "seasonal oral contraceptive pack." What CPT code will be reported for this service?

 • Click **Finish** to return to the Billing and Coding area.
   • Click the exit arrow.
   • Click **Exit the Program** or, if continuing to a new lesson, click **Return to Map** and then click **Yes** on the pop-up menu.

LESSON 7

The Paper Claim CMS-1500

👓 **Reading Assignment:** Chapter 7—The Paper Claim CMS-1500 (08-05)

Patients: Renee Anderson, Louise Parlet, Tristan Tsosie, Jose Imero

Rooms: Reception, Billing and Coding, Check Out

Objectives:

- Identify Mountain View Clinic's policies for verifying a patient's insurance coverage.
- Verify a patient's insurance coverage.
- Determine primary and secondary insurance carriers.
- Identify the subscriber of an insurance plan.
- Prepare documents needed to complete a CMS-1500 claim form.
- Identify general policies and those of Mountain View Clinics related to completion of CMS-1500 claim forms.
- Complete the patient/insured (top) section of the CMS-1500 claim form.
- Use appropriate optical character recognition (OCR) formatting to complete the form.
- Complete the physician/supplier section of the CMS-1500 claim form.

Exercise 1

 Online Activity—Verify Patient's Insurance Coverage

🕐 10 minutes

- Sign in to Mountain View Clinic.
- Select **Renee Anderson** from the patient list.
- Click on **Reception**.
- Click on **Policy** to open the office Policy Manual.
- Using the arrows at the top right of the page, navigate to page 17 and read the section on "Patient Insurance Policies."

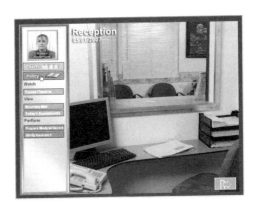

109

1. The Mountain View Clinic Policy Manual expects staff members to obtain and verify correct insurance information upon registration. This will enable the health insurance professional to submit:
   a. a clean claim
   b. a neat claim
   c. more claims per hour
   d. more accurately coded claims.

2. Which of the following actions should be performed during Renee Anderson's insurance verification process? Select all that apply.

   _____ Ask the patient to complete a registration form.

   _____ Ask the patient for her insurance identification card.

   _____ Make a copy of the ID card for the patient record.

   _____ Inform the patient that the entire fee will be due and payable at check-out.

   _____ Inform the patient that she must complete the insurance claim form herself.

   _____ Inform the patient that the copay will be payable at check-out.

 • Click **Close Manual** to return to the Reception area.
• Click on the **Insurance Card**.
• Click on **Ask** next to the question "Do you have insurance?"
• Under View, click on **Insurance Card(s)**.

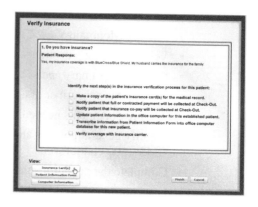

3. Below, verify Ms. Anderson's insurance information by providing the requested information from her insurance card:

Insurance Carrier:

Subscriber:

Plan #:

Group #:

Issue Date:

Copay for PCP:

Copay for Specialist:

- Click **Finish** to return to the Reception area.
- Click the exit arrow.
- Click **Return to Map** and select **Yes** at the pop-up menu to return to the office map.

Exercise 2

Online Activity—Determining Primary and Secondary Carriers

  10 minutes

In this exercise, you'll review the insurance coverage for Louise Parlet and Tristan Tsosie. It is recommended that you select one patient and answer all questions pertinent to that patient in Exercise 2 before proceeding to the next patient.

- Select **Louise Parlet** from the patient list.
- Click on **Billing and Coding**.
- Click on **Charts**.
- Review Ms. Parlet's insurance information as it appears on the Patient Information Form. You can review her insurance cards by clicking the **Patient Information** tab and selecting **2-Insurance Cards**.
- Click **Close Chart** when finished to return to the Billing and Coding area.
- Click the exit arrow.
- Click **Return to Map** and select **Yes** at the pop-up menu to return to the office map.
- Repeat these steps with **Tristan Tsosie**.

1. Below, identify the name of each patient's primary and secondary insurance carriers.

Patient	Primary	Secondary
Louise Parlet		
Tristan Tsosie		

2. For each patient below, identify the name of the subscriber for each plan the patient is enrolled with and note in parentheses the subscriber's relationship to the patient.

Patient	Primary Plan Subscriber (Relationship to Patient)	Secondary Plan Subscriber (Relationship to Patient)
Louise Parlet		
Tristan Tsosie		

Exercise 3

Online Activity—Documents Needed to Complete the CMS-1500 Claim Form

15 minutes

- Select **Renee Anderson** from the patient list.
- Click on **Check Out**.
- Under the Watch heading, click on **Patient Check-Out** and watch the video.
- Click the **X** on the video screen to close the video.
- Click on the **Encounter Form** clipboard.

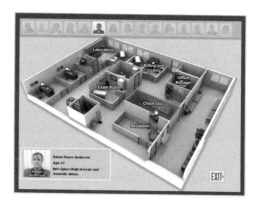

1. Which of the following documents generated during Ms. Anderson's visit will you need for completing the CMS-1500 claim form? Select all that apply.

    _____ Patient Information Form

    _____ Insurance ID Card

    _____ General Health History Questionnaire

    _____ Medication Record

    _____ Encounter Form

    _____ Fee Schedule

2. Below, provide the information that will be obtained from Ms. Anderson's Encounter Form to complete the CMS-1500 form:

Date of Service:

Date of Birth:

Procedures Performed:

Diagnosis:

Diagnosis:

Diagnosis:

• Click **Finish** to return to the Check Out area.
- Click the exit arrow.
- Click **Return to Map** and select **Yes** at the pop-up menu to return to the office map.
- Click on **Billing and Coding**.
- Click on the **Fee Schedule** sheet.

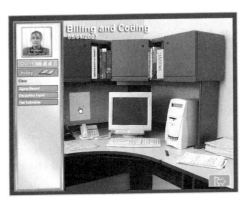

3. In the space below, using Mountain View Clinic's Fee Schedule, itemize the fee for each service performed and verify that the amount indicated as the total amount charged on the Encounter Form is correct so that it can be entered on the CMS-1500 claim form accurately.

 • Click **Finish** to return to the Billing and Coding area.
- Remain in the Billing and Coding area with Renee Anderson as your patient and continue to the next exercise.

Exercise 4

 Online Activity—General Guidelines for Completing the CMS-1500 Claim Form

 10 minutes

- Click on **Policy** to open the office Policy Manual.
- Review all of Mountain View Clinic's policies regarding completion of the CMS-1500 claim form.
- Answer the following questions using the information provided in Mountain View Clinic's Policy Manual.

1. The health insurance professional is responsible for ensuring that the information reported on the CMS-1500 claim form is accurate. According to Mountain View Clinic's Policy Manual (page 34), "submission of a claim for services that were not actually provided" would be considered:
   a. a simple mistake.
   b. a false claim.
   c. a claim with an error.
   d. an incidental error.

2. The Mountain View Clinic Policy Manual (page 34) states that "submission of a claim for services that are not adequately documented in the medical record" could be perceived as:
   a. an oversight.
   b. abusive billing activity.
   c. fraudulent billing activity.
   d. the physician's responsibility.

3. The Mountain View Clinic Policy Manual (page 35) states that when reporting ICD-9 and CPT code information on the CMS-1500 to a health care benefit program, health insurance professionals should be aware that criminal convictions for any health care fraud:
   a. cannot be brought against them because they are just reporting the information provided to them by the physician.
   b. can be brought against them if they knowingly and willfully report information that is incorrect.

4. According to the Mountain View Clinic Policy Manual (pages 40-41), if health insurance professionals are in doubt as to how to report information provided for a particular service on the CMS-1500 claim form, they should:
   a. not submit the claim until they have been told what to do by the physician.
   b. not submit the claim until they have received the appropriate guidance in writing.
   c. submit the claim with the information provided and see whether the claim is denied.
   d. submit the claim with the information provided and refund the money later if necessary.

 • Click **Close Manual** to return to the Billing and Coding area.
   • Remain in the Billing and Coding area with Renee Anderson as your patient and continue to the next exercise.

Exercise 5

 Online Activity—Completing the Patient/Insured Section of the CMS-1500 Claim Form

 20 minutes

• Click on **Charts**.

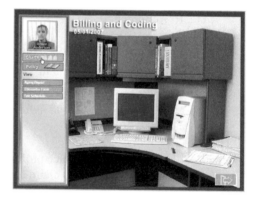

1. Using the correct OCR formatting rules, complete Blocks 1 through 13 of the claim form below. Refer to Ms. Anderson's Patient Information Form and the copy of her insurance card(s).

2. After completing Blocks 1 through 13 of the claim form, double-check the following and explain why you completed the block in the manner that you did.

Block	How Did You Complete?	Explanation
Block 2		
Block 7		
Block 8		

3. The insured's ID number in Block 1a should have been listed as which of the following?
   a. 000-56-3211
   b. 000338888
   c. YLE250011333
   d. YLE-250011333

4. In Block 4, the policy holder's name should be entered as which of the following?
   a. ANDERSON, RENEE
   b. ANDERSON ROBERT
   c. ROBERT ANDERSON
   d. SAME

→ • Leave Ms. Anderson's chart open to continue to the next exercise.

Exercise 6

 Online Activity—Completing the Physician/Supplier Section of the CMS-1500 Claim Form

 20 minutes

• Click on the **Patient Information** tab and select **1-Progress Notes**.

1. Using the information from Ms. Anderson's Progress Notes, complete Blocks 14 through 20 of the claim form below.

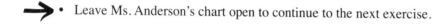

→ • Click **Close Chart** to return to the Billing and Coding area.
   • Click on the **Encounter Form** clipboard and the **Fee Schedule** sheet as needed to complete the following questions.

2. Continue filling Ms. Anderson's claim form by reporting the correct diagnosis codes. The diagnosis information is communicated by the physician to the health insurance specialist on the Encounter Form. Use the diagnosis coding skills that you learned in Lesson 5 to translate the diagnosis information into the correct diagnosis codes and report them in Block 21 below.

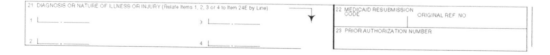

3. Next, you will fill in Block 24 of the claim form. To complete this section, you will need the correct procedural codes. The services are communicated by the physician to the health insurance specialist on the Encounter Form. Use the procedural coding skills that you learned in Lesson 6 to translate the procedural information into the correct procedure codes and report them in Block 24 below.

Using Renee Anderson's Encounter Form and Fee Schedule, also complete Blocks 24A through 24J of the claim form for each service/procedure provided. (*Note:* Do not include services/procedures for which there is no charge. Also, since no provider NPI is provided in Mountain View Clinic's records, use NPI 0002223334 for the attending physician.)

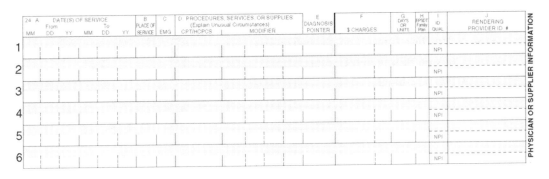

4. Finally, complete Blocks 25 through 33a of the claim form. (*Note:* Use the same date as shown on the Encounter Form. The Clinic NPI is 0001115670.)

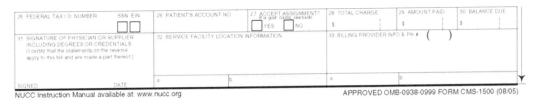

5. Blocks 17 and 17a:
   a. do not need to be completed because the patient is not being referred to Dr. Hayler.
   b. must be completed with Dr. Hayler's name and NPI number.

6. For this claim, the code for Block 24B (place of service) should be:
   a. 11.
   b. 21.
   c. 31.
   d. left blank.

7. In Block 24E, the claim line to report the preventive care service (99396) provided would be linked to which of the following?
   a. V72.31, 611.72, 054.12
   b. V72.31, 611.72
   c. V72.31

8. What should be recorded in Block 24J?
   a. Dr. Hayler's name
   b. Dr. Hayler's NPI number

• Click **Finish** to return to the Billing and Coding area.
• Click the exit arrow.
• Click **Exit the Program** or, if continuing to a new lesson, click **Return to Map** and then click **Yes** on the pop-up menu.

Exercise 7

 Online Activity—Completion of the Entire CMS-1500 Claim Form

 30 minutes

• Select **Jose Imero** from the patient list.
• Click on **Billing and Coding**.
• Click on **Charts**.

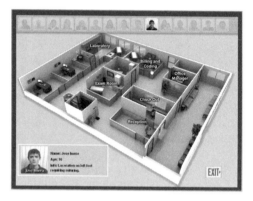

1. Use the source documents in Jose Imero's chart to complete the CMS-1500 claim form below for Jose Imero.

• Click **Close Chart** to return to the Billing and Coding area.
• Click the exit arrow.
• Click **Exit the Program** or, if continuing to a new lesson, click **Return to Map** and then click **Yes** on the pop-up menu.

Electronic Data Interchange: Transactions and Security

✏️ **Reading Assignment:** Chapter 8—Electronic Data Interchange:
Transactions and Security

Patient: Renee Anderson

Room: Billing and Coding

Objectives:

- Demonstrate an understanding of HIPAA requirements for electronic claims submissions using electronic health transaction standards.
- Identify the HIPAA-designated transactions and standard code sets used for insurance claims transmission.
- Understand the use of standard unique identifiers for providers, employers, health plans, and patients as required under HIPAA.
- Compare the CMS-1500 claim form with the electronic claim transmittal form.
- Identify data elements required for electronic claim submissions using format 837P.

Exercise 1

 Online Activity—Understanding HIPAA Requirements for Electronic Claims Using Electronic Health Transaction Standards

 15 minutes

- Sign in to Mountain View Clinic.
- Select **Renee Anderson** from the patient list.
- Click on **Billing and Coding**.
- Click on **Policy** to open the office Policy Manual.
- Type "transaction standards" in the search bar and click once on the magnifying glass.
- Read the section of the Policy Manual on transaction standards at Mountain View Clinic.

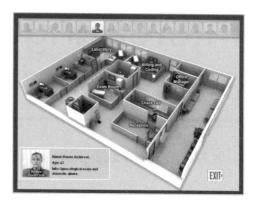

1. What HIPAA Administrative Simplification rules and standards does Mountain View Clinic adhere to in an effort to standardize the exchange of health care electronically?
   a. Electronic Health Transaction Standards
   b. Standard Code Sets
   c. Unique Identifiers for Providers, Employers, Health Plans, and Patients
   d. All of the above

2. Electronic Health Transaction Standards are guidelines that govern how information is

   _____ between computer systems for eligibility verification, claims, etc.

3. Indicate whether each of the following statements related to HIPAA's requirements for electronic claim submission is true or false.

   a. _____ Mountain View Clinic has 15 employees: 12 are full-time and 3 are part-time employees. According to Medicare, the clinic is not required to send claims electronically in the HIPAA format and may continue to submit paper claims.

   b. _____ A benefit of electronic claims submission is quicker reimbursement from payers.

   c. _____ Electronic claims submission has proven to reduce office expenses.

   d. _____ Demographic information does not have to be entered into electronic billing software systems.

   e. _____ When submitting claims electronically, the provider has an accurate and detailed audit trail showing what was submitted and accepted by the insurance company.

→ • Keep the Policy Manual open to continue to the next exercise.

Exercise 2

Online Activity—Identifying the Transactions and Standard Code Sets Used for Insurance Claims Transmission

  10 minutes

- Continue to review the transaction standards in the office Policy Manual.

1. What are standard code sets?

2. The designated standard codes sets that will be used by Mountain View Clinic are

   _____ and _____ codes.

3. Mountain View Clinic collects and records data elements that are required under HIPAA Transaction Code Standards on the Patient Information Form in the chart. Using your textbook for reference, identify which of these are required elements? Select all that apply.

   _____ Patient account number

   _____ Emergency contact

   _____ Relationship to patient

   _____ Patient telephone number

   _____ Patient signature

   _____ Insurance address

→ • Keep the Policy Manual open and continue to the next exercise.

Exercise 3

Online Activity—Understanding the Use of Standard Unique Identifiers for Providers, Employers, Health Plans, and Patients

15 minutes

• Continue to review the transaction standards in the office Policy Manual.

1. Standard unique identifiers are unique alphanumeric codes that facilitate electronic transactions and are assigned to which of the following?
   a. Providers
   b. Employers
   c. Health plans
   d. Patients
   e. All of the above

2. The _____ is an all-numeric 10-character number assigned to providers to be used in transactions with all health plans.

3. An _____ is used to identify employers when submitting claims.

4. Indicate whether each of the following statements is true or false.

   a. _____ Standard unique identifiers for health plans that process and pay electronic health care transactions were issued in April of 2010.

   b. _____ Standard unique identifiers for patients are currently "on hold."

 • Click **Close Manual** to return to the Billing and Coding area.
   • Click on the **Encounter Form** clipboard.

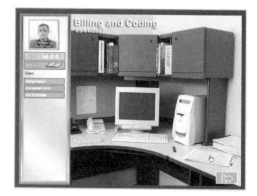

5. What is Mountain View Clinic's Federal Tax ID # or EIN? _____

6. How do employers use a standard unique employer identification number (EIN)?
   (**Hint:** You may need to return to the office Policy Manual and search again for "transaction standards" to find this information.)

- Click **Finish** to return to the Billing and Coding area.
- Click the exit arrow.
- Click **Exit the Program** or, if continuing to a new lesson, click **Return to Map** and then click **Yes** on the pop-up menu.

Exercise 4

 Writing Activity—Comparing the CMS-1500 Claim Form with the Electronic Claim Transmittal Format 837P

 20 minutes

- Refer to the printed forms from Lesson 7, Exercises 5 and 6, in which you completed a CMS-1500 claim form for Renee Anderson.

 1. Using the information provided in your textbook (see Table 8.5), indicate where the identified information from Renee Anderson's claim form (column 1) would be located on the CMS-1500 claim form (column 2) in comparison with the electronic claim transmittal form 837P (column 3).

Information on Renee Anderson's Claim Form	CMS-1500 Box #	837P Data Element #
ANDERSON RENEE		
ANDERSON ROBERT		
YLE250011333		
MONTROSE AND ASSOCIATES LAW FIRM		
V72.31		
99396		
123456789		

2. The patient's gender would be identified in data element # _____ on the electronic claim transmittal form 837P.

3. The patient's relationship to the insured would be identified in data element # _____ on the electronic claim transmittal form 837P.

4. The physician's signature would be identified in Block # _____ of the CMS-1500 claim form.

5. The physician's NPI number would be identified in Block # _____ of the CMS-1500 claim form.

6. Using the information provided in your textbook (see Table 8.6), indicate whether the information identified is a required or situational data element when submitting electronic claims using the HIPAA standard 837P electronic claim transmittal form.

Description of Data Element	**Type of Data Element**
_____ Patient date of birth (data element #1251)	a. Required
_____ Subscriber address line (data element #166)	b. Situational
_____ Auto accident (data element #1362)	
_____ Patient's or authorized person's signature (data element #1351)	
_____ Date of LMP (data element #1251)	
_____ CPT code (data element #234)	
_____ CPT modifier (data element #1339)	
_____ Signature of physician (data element #1073)	
_____ Physician's NPI (data element #127)	

Receiving Payments and Insurance Problem Solving

 Reading Assignment: Chapter 9—Receiving Payments and Insurance Problem Solving

Patients: Renee Anderson, Jose Imero

Rooms: Check Out, Billing and Coding, Reception

Objectives:

- Discuss health insurance payment policies
- Follow the claims process
- Understand the components of the Explanation of Benefits (EOB) form.
- Recording the daily payment transactions.

Exercise 1

 Online Activity—Health Insurance Claim Filing and Payment Policies

20 minutes

- Sign in to Mountain View Clinic
- Select **Renee Anderson** from the patient list.
- Click on **Check Out**.
- Click on **Policy** to open the office Policy Manual
- Read the Financial Policy beginning on page 32 of the Mountain View Policy Manual and complete the following statements regarding collection of payments and copays.

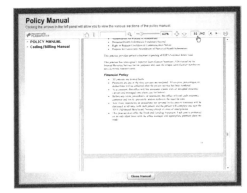

1. The office will file insurance claims with _____ insurance carriers and managed care organizations.

2. Payments are due _____ _____ _____ services are rendered.

3. All copay, percentage, or deductible payments will be collected _____ the patient's service has been rendered.

4. To ensure payment of claims, this office will call each insurance company and

_____, _____, and/or _____ any visits, procedures or treatment to patients.

5. Any visits, treatments or procedures not covered by the patient's insurance will be discussed in advance with each patient and patients will complete and sign the

_____ _____ _____ advising the patient that they will be responsible for payment of the service.

- Click **Close Manual** to return to the Check Out desk.
- Click on **Charts**.
- Click on the **Patient Information** tab and select **1-Patient Information Form** or **2-Insurance Cards** to answer the following questions.

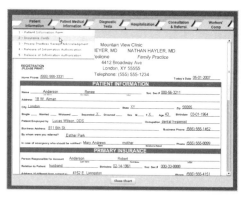

6. Answer the following true and false questions that will affect the claim filing and payment of Renee Anderson's visit to Mountain View Clinic.

    a. _____ Mountain View Clinic participates with Renee Anderson's insurance.

    b. _____ The copay due for services provided to Renee Anderson at the time of service is $15.

    c. _____ According to the assignment of benefits signed by Renee Anderson, the insurance payment for services provided will be sent directly to her.

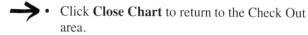

- Click **Close Chart** to return to the Check Out area.
- Under the Watch heading, click on **Patient Check-Out** and watch the video.

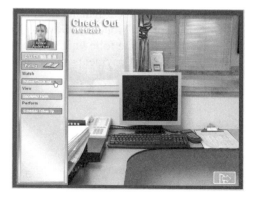

7. Indicate whether the following statement is true or false.

_____   Renee Anderson's copay was successfully collected by Mountain View Clinic at the time of service.

→ • Click the **X** on the video screen to close the video.
• Click the exit arrow.
• Click **Return to Map** and select **Yes** at the pop-up menu to return to the office map.
• Select **Jose Imero** from the patient list.
• Click on **Check Out**.
• Click on **Charts**.
• Click on the **Patient Information** tab and select **1-Patient Information Form** or **2-Insurance Cards** to answer the following questions.

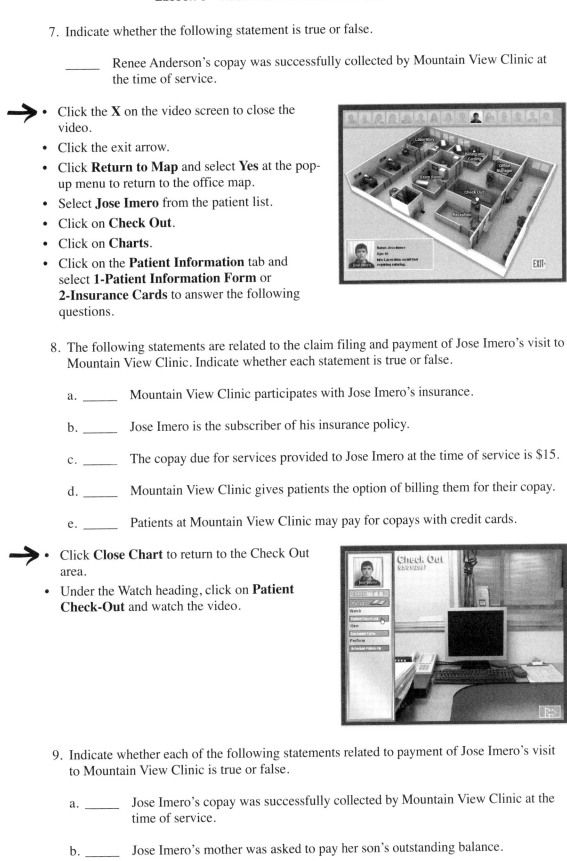

8. The following statements are related to the claim filing and payment of Jose Imero's visit to Mountain View Clinic. Indicate whether each statement is true or false.

a. _____   Mountain View Clinic participates with Jose Imero's insurance.

b. _____   Jose Imero is the subscriber of his insurance policy.

c. _____   The copay due for services provided to Jose Imero at the time of service is $15.

d. _____   Mountain View Clinic gives patients the option of billing them for their copay.

e. _____   Patients at Mountain View Clinic may pay for copays with credit cards.

→ • Click **Close Chart** to return to the Check Out area.
• Under the Watch heading, click on **Patient Check-Out** and watch the video.

9. Indicate whether each of the following statements related to payment of Jose Imero's visit to Mountain View Clinic is true or false.

a. _____   Jose Imero's copay was successfully collected by Mountain View Clinic at the time of service.

b. _____   Jose Imero's mother was asked to pay her son's outstanding balance.

c. _____   Jose Imero's previous balance was successfully collected by Mountain View Clinic at this service.

10. Jose's mother was asked to pay an outstanding balance on her son's account. Explain what you think was done incorrectly at Jose's previous visit.

• Click the **X** on the video screen to close the video.
• Click the exit arrow.
• Click **Return to Map** and select **Yes** at the pop-up menu to return to the office map.

Exercise 2

 Online Activity—Following the Claims Process

 15 minutes

• Select **Renee Anderson** from the patient list.
• Click on **Billing and Coding**.
• Click on **Charts**.

1. Let's assume that Ms. Anderson's health insurance company has not responded to a claim that was filed on her behalf. Indicate whether each of the following statements about the claim process is true or false.

   a. _____ The health insurance professional will need to contact Blue Cross/Blue Shield to follow up on Renee Anderson's claim.

   b. _____ The health insurance professional should automatically rebill the claim if there has been no response from the insurance carrier within 30 days.

   c. _____ Claim correction forms can be used to follow up on claims if it is determined that an error has been made in billing.

   d. _____ If the claim has been denied and the health insurance specialist does not agree with the denial, the bill must be written off.

   e. _____ If the health insurance specialist is concerned that the insurance carrier is not abiding by the terms of their contract, the specialist can contact the State Insurance Commission for assistance.

2. The health insurance specialist should have a mechanism in place to track Ms. Anderson's claim if it is determined that the claim is not processed by the insurance carrier:
   a. within a week from claim submission.
   b. within 3 weeks from claim submission.
   c. within 4-6 weeks from claim submission.
   d. within 2-3 months from claim submission.

3. In the event that Ms. Anderson's claim is not processed promptly and an inquiry to her insurance carrier is required to determine the status of the unpaid claim, what would be the most efficient and most effective method for the health insurance professional to handle the follow-up?
   a. Contact the carrier by phone
   b. Resubmit the claim
   c. Fax a follow-up claim to the carrier
   d. Copy a system-generated report of unpaid claims and send it to the carrier

4. In the event that Ms. Anderson's claim is processed and the Explanation of Benefits has denied the claim, the health insurance professional should:
   a. record the denial and bill the patient.
   b. review the EOB to determine why the claim was denied and confirm its legitimacy.
   c. immediately appeal the claim.
   d. write off the service that is denied.

- Click **Close Chart** to return to the Billing and Coding area.
- Click the exit arrow.
- Click **Return to Map** and select **Yes** at the pop-up menu to return to the office map.
- Keep Renee Anderson as your patient and continue to the next exercise.

Exercise 3

 Online Activity—Components of the Explanation of Benefits (EOB) Form

30 minutes

- Click on **Reception**.
- Click on the **Stackable Trays**.
- Click the number **6** to examine that piece of mail.
- Answer the following questions while reviewing the Explanation of Benefits form.

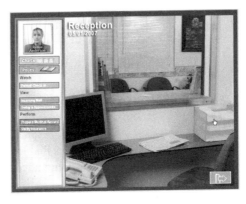

1. The EOB form is for services provided to _____ _____, a patient at Mountain View Clinic.

2. The EOB is from _____, the patient's insurance carrier.

3. Indicate whether each of the following statements regarding interpretation of an EOB is true or false.

   a. _____ It is not important for the health insurance specialist to know whether the practice is participating with the insurance carrier who has sent the EOB form that the specialist is interpreting.

b. _____ According to information previously reviewed in the Mountain View Clinic Policy Manual, the practice is participating with the patient's insurance carrier.

c. _____ Participating insurance agreements generally limit the amount that the patient can be billed through an established reimbursement schedule.

4. According to the EOB, on what date did the patient receive the service?
a. 3/5/2007
b. 3/9/2007
c. 4/25/2007
d. 4/28/2007

5. According to the EOB, on what date did the insurance carrier receive the claim?
a. 3/5/2007
b. 3/9/2007
c. 4/25/2007
d. 4/28/2007

6. According to the EOB, on what date was the claim processed by the insurance carrier?
a. 3/5/2007
b. 3/9/2007
c. 4/25/2007
d. 4/28/2007

7. According to the EOB, what was the patient's ID number?
a. EXCTJG123456
b. 307890765
c. 98700
d. 99205

8. According to the EOB, what number was assigned to this claim by the insurance carrier?
a. EXCTJG123456
b. 307890765
c. 98700
d. 99205

9. The EOB indicates that Dr. _____ is the physician who provided the services and is being advised of the benefits that will be paid for this claim.

10. The services that are being explained on the EOB are designated by the CPT code

_____.

11. According to the EOB, the total amount charged by Mountain View Clinic for this service

was _____.

12. The EOB indicates that the amount paid to the provider by the insurance carrier is

_____.

13. The EOB indicates that the patient is responsible for paying $_____ to Mountain View Clinic.

14. Explain why there is a write-off amount of $20 indicated on the Explanation of Benefits.

15. Let's assume that upon receipt of the EOB for this patient, the health insurance professional determines that the insurance company has downcoded the claim. This means:
    a. the insurance carrier has denied the claim based on the diagnosis submitted.
    b. the insurance carrier does not recognize the CPT code submitted.
    c. the insurance carrier has assigned a substitute code (one that the carrier believes fits the service performed) at a lower level than reported.
    d. the insurance carrier has requested additional information from the provider.

16. In the event that the EOB indicates a downcoding by the insurance carrier, the health insurance professional should:
    a. write off the unpaid balance by the insurance carrier.
    b. bill the patient for any unpaid balance by the insurance carrier.
    c. change coding techniques based on the carrier's interpretation of them.
    d. contact the claims adjuster and ask the reason for downcoding.

17. If the EOB for the patient indicates that the claim has been denied because it was not filed within the time limit set by the insurance carrier, the health insurance professional should immediately:
    a. appeal the claim.
    b. bill the patient.
    c. write off the service.
    d. examine the practice's contract with the insurance carrier to confirm timely filing guidelines and contact the carrier to determine whether there are any allowances for late filing of claims that may be relevant.

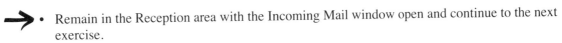

• Remain in the Reception area with the Incoming Mail window open and continue to the next exercise.

Exercise 4

Online Activity—Recording the Daily Payment Transactions

 20 minutes

- Click the numbers or arrows at the top of the Incoming Mail window to examine and read each piece of mail.

1. A daysheet will be used to post all payments that were received in the incoming mail. Post all payments received on 5/1/07 on the daysheet on the next page.

2. According to the daysheet prepared for 5/1/07, the total amount of payments that will be deposited in the bank is _____.

3. According to the daysheet prepared for 5/1/07, the total amount of contractual write-offs was _____.

4. A personal check returned due to insufficient funds should be posted on the daysheet in the column labeled _____ since it is a charge, rather than a payment.

5. When posting a check returned due to insufficient funds, it is important to also post the returned check _____, which is an additional amount charged by the bank.

 • Click **Finish** to return to the Reception area.
- Click the exit arrow.
- Click **Exit the Program** or, if continuing to a new lesson, click **Return to Map** and then click **Yes** on the pop-up menu.

Mountain View Clinic
Daysheet

Date	Professional Service	Fee	Payment	Adjustment	New Balance	Old Balance	Patient's Name	Distribution	
								Dr. Hayler	Dr. Meyer

TOTALS

TOTALS

LESSON 10

Office and Insurance Collection Strategies

📖 **Reading Assignment:** Chapter 10—Office and Insurance Collection Strategies

Patient: Jesus Santo

Rooms: Billing and Coding, Reception

Objectives:

- Understand office collection policies.
- Understand the types of fee adjustments available to patients.
- Understand ways to determine fees and describe an office's fee policies.
- Review an aging report.
- Understand the process for handling returned checks.

Exercise 1

 Online Activity—Understanding Office Collection Policies

 15 minutes

- Sign in to Mountain View Clinic.
- Select **Jesus Santo** from the patient list.
- Click on **Billing and Coding**.
- Click on **Policy** to open the office Policy Manual.
- Keep the Policy Manual open as you answer the following questions.

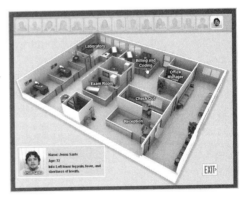

1. In Mountain View Clinic's Policy Manual, the section titled "Telephone Policy" states that patients should be reminded that any payment due is expected:
   a. before the scheduled appointment.
   b. at the time the service is rendered.
   c. within 30 days after the service is provided.
   d. within 60 days after the service is provided.

2. In Mountain View Clinic's Policy Manual, the "Patient Insurance Policy" states that if a patient does not have insurance coverage, the patient should be advised of the charges when the appointment is made and provided with a detailed statement of all charges after services have been provided. A detailed statement of charges could be provided to the patient with a copy of the:
   a. Assignment of Benefits Form.
   b. Patient Information Form.
   c. Encounter Form.
   d. Progress Note.

 3. Indicate whether each of the following statements is true or false, based on Mountain View Clinic's office collection policies and information provided in the textbook.

   a. _____ Mountain View Clinic sends out patient statements at the end of each month.

   b. _____ An advantage of cycle billing is that is helps the office staff handle incoming telephone calls about billing.

   c. _____ Jesus Santo would receive a statement on the 30th of the month.

   d. _____ The patient receives his or her first billing statement after 30 days (from date of service).

   e. _____ The patient's account is first considered overdue at 60 days.

   f. _____ The most effective way to add a dun message is to write the message by hand directly on the statement.

   g. _____ The health insurance professional would be expected to contact the patient by telephone when the patient's account is more than 60 days overdue.

   h. _____ If the patient has not paid his or her bill by 120 days from the date of service, the account will be turned over to a collection agency.

   i. _____ Patients who have insurance will not receive a statement until the insurance carrier has processed the claim.

4. Which of the following are appropriate guidelines that Mountain View Clinic can use to determine when an account should be turned over for collection? Select all that apply.

_____ When patients state that they will not pay or there is a denial of responsibility.

_____ When delinquency coexists with marital problems, divorce proceedings, or child support agreements.

_____ When the office does not have the time to follow up on patient accounts on its own.

_____ When patients give false information.

_____ When patients break their promise to pay.

_____ When patients say they do not have the money to pay and the office determines that the collection agency can expedite payment.

_____ When patients suggest that they might be reimbursed by their insurance company if they file the claim themselves.

➡ • Keep the Policy Manual open and continue to the next exercise.

Exercise 2

  Online Activity—Understanding the Types of Fee Adjustments Available to Patients

🕐 20 minutes

• In the office Policy Manual, type "related issues" in the search bar and click on the magnifying glass.

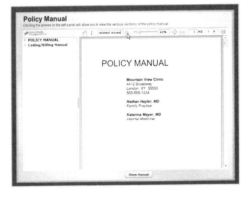

1. One of the physicians at Mountain View clinic plays golf with Dr. Smith every Saturday. Is it appropriate for the clinic to grant a professional courtesy adjustment to Dr. Smith's office visit?
   a. Yes, this is referred to as a professional courtesy and is allowed in all cases.
   b. No, this could be a violation of the Medicare Anti-Kickback statute and HIPAA fraud and abuse laws.

2. An interim rule from the Centers for Medicare and Medicaid Services (CMS), published in the Federal Register dated July 24, 2004, identifies proper ways for the medical office or practice (the "entity") to offer professional courtesy adjustments. Which of the following are examples of proper procedures? Select all that apply.

_____   The professional courtesy is offered if a physician has a close relationship with another physician.

_____   The professional courtesy is offered to all physicians on the entity's bona fide medical staff without regard to volume or value of referrals or other business generated between parties.

_____   The entity's professional courtesy policy is written and approved in advance by the entity's governing body.

_____   The professional courtesy is offered to any member of the clergy.

_____   The entity makes the decision to add this to its Policy Manual.

3. The practice of submitting a charge to the patient's insurance company and, at the same time, writing off the patient's coinsurance amount is referred to as:
   a. professional courtesy.
   b. insurance only.
   c. small-balance write-off.
   d. same-day write-off.

4. Which of the following is correct if the patient's contractual obligation with the insurance company requires him or her to pay a copay or coinsurance? Select all that apply.

_____   The billing office may waive copayments at its discretion.

_____   The billing office must attempt to collect the copayment or coinsurance.

_____   Waiving of the copayment could violate the contract between the patient and the insurance company.

_____   Waiving of the copayment could violate the contract between the insurance company and the patient's employer.

_____   Waiving of the copayment could violate the contract between the physician and the insurance company.

5. According to Mountain View Clinic's Policy Manual, if a biller determines that an entire charge needs to be written off a patient's account, they should contact

_____ _____ _____ for assistance.

6. A medical office determines that it will cost the practice more to collect a balance of $1.10 than it is worth. This type of write-off is known as a _____ _____

_____.

→ • Keep the Policy Manual open and continue to the next exercise.

Exercise 3

 Online Activity—Understanding Ways to Determine Fees and Describe an Office's Fee Policies

 20 minutes

- Continue reviewing the Policy Manual's discussion under "Related Issues."

 1. Indicate whether each of the following statements regarding fees is true or false based on Mountain View Clinic's Policy Manual and the information provided in the textbook.

    a. _____ Mountain View Clinic's Fee Schedule is a list of accepted charges and established allowances for specific medical procedures.

    b. _____ Mountain View Clinic's fees were developed based on prevailing norms and input from their patients.

    c. _____ According to Mountain View Clinic's policy, self-pay patients are entitled to the "lowest fee schedule" the office has.

    d. _____ It is not required that Mountain View Clinic make its Fee Schedule available to patients.

    e. _____ Once fee schedules are established, routine discounting of charges may still occur.

    f. _____ If a discount is offered, it must be applied to the total fee, not just the portion that is paid by the patient.

    g. _____ All discounts to fees must be posted to the patient's financial record with the reason or circumstances documented.

 - Click **Close Manual** to return to the Billing and Coding area.
- Click on the **Encounter Form** clipboard and **Fee Schedule** sheet as needed to complete the following questions.

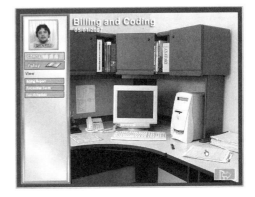

2. Complete the chart below by listing the services that were performed for Mr. Santo. (*Note:* Use the Encounter Form to complete the left column; use the Fee Schedule for the right column.)

Services Performed	Fee Schedule Amount

3. Mr. Santo's total charges were $210.00, which he paid in full with cash at the time of service. Could Mountain View Clinic have offered Mr. Santo a cash discount? Why or why not?

4. If Mr. Santo had indicated financial hardship, Mountain View Clinic could have offered a hardship waiver. Which of the following statements about hardship waivers is (are) true? Select all that apply.

_____ Financial hardship waivers are limited by the federal government to no more than 10% of the entire bill.

_____ Financial hardship waivers can vary from 24% to 100% of the bill.

_____ A copy of the patient's wage and tax statement should be reviewed to determine financial hardship.

_____ The reason for the fee reduction must be documented in the patient's medical record.

_____ It is not necessary to provide financial hardship consistently among patients.

_____ The practice should develop a written policy related to financial hardship.

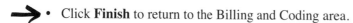 • Click **Finish** to return to the Billing and Coding area.

• Remain in the Billing and Coding area with Jesus Santo as your patient and continue to the next exercise.

Exercise 4

Online Activity—Reviewing an Aging Report

 15 minutes

- Click on the **Aging Report** sheet.

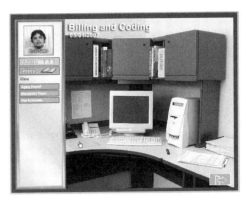

1. Age analysis is done by systematically arranging the aging report in what order?
   a. Arranged in order by the date of the first statement sent.
   b. Arranged in order by the date of the last statement sent.
   c. Arranged in order by the date of service.
   d. Arranged in order based on the age of the treating provider.

2. Accounts are usually aged in time periods of:
   a. 10, 20, 30, and 40 days.
   b. 10, 30, 60, and 90 days.
   c. 30, 60, 90, and 120 days.
   d. 30, 60, 80, and 120 days.

3. Which patient listed on the aging report has insurance coverage through his wife, who is the subscriber of the plan?
   a. Jacob Abraham
   b. Frank Bullock
   c. Larry Nerod
   d. Emanual Perez

4. Which patient listed on the aging report has sent a payment most recently?
   a. Jacob Abraham
   b. Frank Bullock
   c. Cynthia Dearing
   d. Larry Nerod

5. Which patient listed on the aging report has the largest amount due to Mountain View Clinic?
   a. Jacob Abraham
   b. Frank Bullock
   c. Kirsha Macken
   d. Emanual Perez

6. Which patient listed on the aging report has the oldest account (over 120 days old)?
   a. Frank Bullock
   b. Cynthia Dearing
   c. Kirsha Macken
   d. Larry Nerod

7. If a patient does not make a payment to his or her account within 120 days from the date of service, Mountain View Clinic's policy is to:
   a. make a telephone call to the patient requesting payment within 7-10 days.
   b. turn the account over to a collection agency.
   c. write off the balance of the bill as an uncollectible debt.
   d. file a small claims suite for the delinquent account.

8. What percentage of the total accounts receivable is over 120 days old?
   a. 16.18%
   b. 49.30%
   c. 15.10%
   d. 19.41%

9. Of the following patients, which three have claims that require the most immediate attention by the health insurance professional? Select the three that apply and be prepared to explain the reasoning for your selections.

   _____ Jacob Abraham

   _____ Frank Bullock

   _____ Cynthia Dearing

   _____ Kirsha Macken

   _____ Larry Nerod

   _____ Emanual Perez

10. Based on Mountain View Clinic's collection policy, what actions should have already been taken by the health insurance professional for collection of the three claims you identified in the previous question?

11. When calling patients to make credit arrangements and to establish a payment plan, it is important for the health insurance professional to keep in mind that an installment plan of more than four payments is subject to the regulations set by the Federal Truth in Lending Act of 1968, which requires that the payee (in this case, the medical office) disclose:
    a. any monthly finance charges.
    b. the date when payments are due.
    c. the amount of any late-payment charges.
    d. all of the above.

12. Why do you think it is important for the health insurance professional to review the aging report?

- Click **Finish** to return to the Billing and Coding area.
- Click the exit arrow.
- Click **Return to Map** and select **Yes** at the pop-up menu to return to the office map.
- Keep Jesus Santo as your patient and continue to the next exercise.

Exercise 5

Online Activity—Understanding the Process for Handling Returned Checks

 10 minutes

- Click on **Reception**.
- Click on the **Stackable Trays** to view today's incoming mail.
- Click the number **7** to examine that piece of mail.

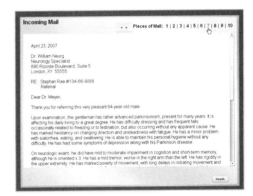

1. What does NSF stand for?

2. What was the amount of the bank's fee charged to Mountain View Clinic's account?

3. Of the following choices, select the three most appropriate and effective actions that the health insurance professional at Mountain View Clinic can take when a payment made by check is returned by the patient's bank because of nonsufficient funds.

_____ Simply redeposit the check.

_____ Contact the patient immediately by phone about the situation.

_____ Contact the bank to determine whether there are currently sufficient funds in the account so that the check can be redeposited.

_____ Repost the check amount to the patient's account, and allow the additional charge to bill on his or her monthly statement.

_____ Send the patient a certified letter (with return receipt requested), notifying the patient of the NSF check and the patient's obligations.

4. Can the clinic charge a penalty for a returned check? If so, explain how the patient should be notified of such a charge.

 • Click **Finish** to return to the Reception area.
 • Click the exit arrow.
 • Click **Exit the Program** or, if continuing to a new lesson, click **Return to Map** and then click **Yes** on the pop-up menu.

LESSON 11

Blue Cross/Blue Shield, Private Insurance, and Managed Care Plans

Reading Assignment: Chapter 11—The Blue Plans, Private Insurance, and Managed Care Plans

Patients: Teresa Hernandez, Tristan Tsosie, Jose Imero, Louse Parlet, Jade Wong, John R. Simmons

Room: Billing and Coding

Objectives:

• Identify Blue Cross/Blue Shield (BCBS), private insurance, and managed care plans.
• Identify and compare deductibles and prior authorization requirements for various insurance plans.
• Identify and compare various copayments and method of collection of copays.
• Identify the procedure for obtaining authorizations for medical services, tests, and procedures.
• Complete a claim form for a patient with Blue Cross/Blue Shield as secondary coverage.
• Complete a claim form for a patient with private insurance coverage.

Exercise 1

Online Activity—Identifying and Comparing Characteristics of Different Types of Insurance Plans

  20 minutes

• Sign in to Mountain View Clinic.
• Before selecting a patient, read question 1 of this exercise. Then follow the steps below to find the information required. Fill in each patient's portion of the question as you go (or take notes!).
• Select **Teresa Hernandez** from the patient list.
• Click on **Billing and Coding**.
• Click on **Charts**.

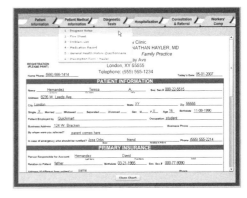

- Review the patient's insurance information as it appears on the Patient Information Form. (*Note:* If applicable, you can also review the patient's insurance cards by clicking on the **Patient Information** tab and selecting **Insurance Cards**.)
- Click **Close Chart** to return to the Billing and Coding area.
- Click the exit arrow.
- Click **Return to Map** and select **Yes** at the pop-up menu to return to the office map.
- Repeat the previous steps for the following patients: **Louise Parlet**, **Tristan Tsosie**, **Jose Imero**, **Jade Wong**, **John Simmons**, and **Hu Huang**.

1. Which of the following patients have primary insurance coverage through a Blue Cross/Blue Shield plan, a private insurance plan, or a managed care plan? Select all that apply.

_____ Teresa Hernandez

_____ Louise Parlet

_____ Tristan Tsosie

_____ Jose Imero

_____ Jade Wong

_____ John Simmons

_____ Hu Huang

 - For the remaining questions in this exercise (2 through 4) and questions 1 and 2 in Exercise 2, you will follow the same set of steps for **Louise Parlet**, **Tristan Tsosie**, and **Jose Imero**. It is recommended that you select one patient and answer all questions pertinent to that patient before proceeding to the next patient.
- Select **Louise Parlet** from the patient list.
- Click on **Billing and Coding**.
- Click on **Charts**.
- Click on the **Patient Information** tab and select **Insurance Cards**.

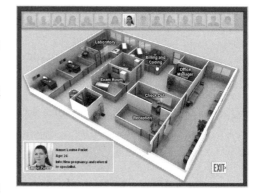

2. For each patient listed below, identify the amount of the annual deductible the patient is responsible for under his or her primary insurance plan, as indicated on the patient's insurance card.

Patient	Annual Deductible
Louise Parlet	
Tristan Tsosie	
Jose Imero	

3. Identify whether each of the following patients has a preferred provider organization (PPO) or a health maintenance organization (HMO) for his or her primary insurance plan, as indicated on the patient's insurance card. Place an "X" under the heading that applies for each patient.

Patient	PPO	HMO
Louise Parlet		
Tristan Tsosie		
Jose Imero		

4. Identify which of the following patients' primary insurance cards indicate that prior authorization is required before hospital admission. Place an "X" in the right-hand column for any patient whose insurance requires this.

Patient	Prior Authorization Required for Hospitalization
Louise Parlet	
Tristan Tsosie	
Jose Imero	

• Remain in the Billing and Coding area with your current patient's chart open and continue to Exercise 2.

Exercise 2

Online Activity—Identification and Collection of Copayments

20 minutes

1. Below, record the different copay amounts required by each of the listed patients' primary insurance plans when the patient sees a primary care provider and when the patient sees a specialist. (*Reminder:* You will find this information on each patient's insurance card.)

Patient	Primary Care Provider Copay	Specialist Copay
Louise Parlet		
Tristan Tsosie		
Jose Imero		

• Click **Close Chart** to return to the Billing and Coding area.

• Click on the **Encounter Form** clipboard and **Charts** as needed to complete the following questions.

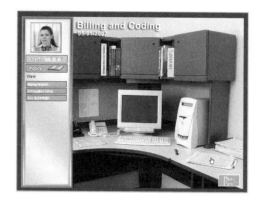

2. Identify the amount of copay due from the following patients for their visit to see one of the primary care physicians at Mountain View Clinic. Also indicate whether or not the copay was collected (and the amount collected) at the time of the visit.

Patient	Amount of Copay Due for Patient's Primary Insurance	Amount Collected for Copay at Time of Visit
Louise Parlet		
Tristan Tsosie		
Jose Imero		

• Click the exit arrow.

• Click **Return to Map** and select **Yes** at the pop-up menu to return to the office map

• Select **Louise Parlet** from the patient list.

• Click on **Check Out**.

• Click on **Policy** to open the office Policy Manual.

• Find answers to the following questions about copayments by using the Policy Manual search bar. (**Hint:** Search for the terms "copay" and "co-pay.")

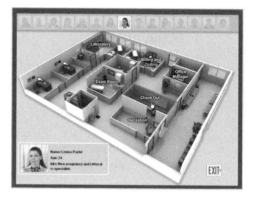

3. When should patients of Mountain View Clinic be reminded that copayment is due at the time service is rendered?
   a. When they schedule an appointment
   b. When they check in
   c. When they check out
   d. When the clinic sends them a bill for the outstanding charge

4. According to the Mountain View Clinic Policy Manual, collection of copays at the time of service is the responsibility of:
   a. scheduling staff.
   b. check-in staff.
   c. check-out staff.
   d. billing staff.

5. During Jose Imero's visit, the receptionist explains that it is Mountain View Clinic's policy to collect copays at the time of service. Why is it important that copayments are collected at the time of service?

 • Click **Close Manual** to return to the Check Out area.
   • Remain in the Check Out area with Louise Parlet as your patient and continue to the next exercise.

Exercise 3

 Online Activity—Obtaining Precertification and Authorization for Medical Service Referrals, Tests, or Procedures

 20 minutes

   • Under the Watch heading, click on **Patient Check Out** and watch the video.

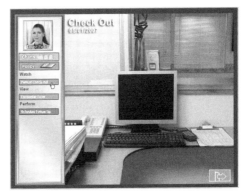

1. What is Louise Parlet's diagnosis that leads to a referral for services?

2. To whom does Dr. Hayler refer Ms. Parlet?

3. What indicator on Louise Parlet's primary insurance card would alert the check-out staff that precertification may be required for a referral to an obstetrician?
   a. Copay
   b. Group #
   c. Employer name
   d. PPO

4. What statement is on the back of Louise Parlet's insurance card with Teachers' Health Group that indicates precertification may be required for a referral to an obstetrician?
   a. "Certain services may require preauthorization."
   b. "To locate a preferred provider, call the phone number indicated."
   c. Neither a nor b is written on the back of the card.
   d. Both a and b are written on the back of the card.

5. Louise Parlet assumes that both of her insurance providers will cover the referred services that Dr. Lockett will provide. Why should the Mountain View Clinic staff call her insurance providers to verify coverage of Dr. Lockett's services?
   a. Mountain View Clinic will not get paid for today's services if the insurance providers are not contacted.
   b. There is no need to verify coverage; it is safe to assume.
   c. There is no need to verify coverage; it is the responsibility of Dr. Lockett's office.
   d. Verifying this information complies with the practice's mission statement and the practice's Policy Manual to arrange referrals and to provide the highest professional care and patient satisfaction.

6. The office staff member asks whether the physician Ms. Parlet is being referred to is an "in-network provider." If Dr. Lockett is an in-network provider, this means:
   a. Dr. Locket is within driving distance from Mountain View Clinic.
   b. Dr. Locket is a participating physician with the patient's insurance plan and out-of-pocket expenses will be less for the patient.
   c. Dr. Lockett is a participating physician with the patient's insurance plan and the provider will pay the patient directly.
   d. Dr. Lockett is employed by Teachers' Health Group so there will be an out-of-pocket discount for the patient.

7. Which of the following steps are performed by the medical assistant to obtain authorization for a referral to a specialist? Select all that apply.

   _____ A telephone call is made to Teachers' Health Group.

   _____ A telephone call is made to Blue Cross/Blue Shield.

   _____ A fax is sent to Teachers' Health Group to obtain precertification.

   _____ A verification number is obtained from Teachers' Health Group.

   _____ The medical assistant asks Teachers' Health Group if Dr. Lockett is an "in-network" provider.

   _____ The medical assistant requests Teachers' Health Group to fax the completed precertification form.

   _____ The medical assistant asks Blue Cross/Blue Shield to schedule Ms. Parlet's appointment with Dr. Lockett.

8. If Dr. Lockett is not a participating provider with either Teachers' Health Group or Blue Cross/Blue Shield, which of the following is not an option open to Ms. Parlet?
   a. She can request the name(s) of participating obstetric providers in the area that do contract with either or both of her insurance plans.
   b. She can accept treatment from an out-of-network provider and pay a higher copay, according to the rules of her plan.
   c. She can accept treatment from an out-of-network provider and request a discount from the provider known as "insurance only" billing.
   d. She can opt to pay the charges herself.

 • Click the **X** to close the video.
   • Click the exit arrow.
   • Click **Return to Map** and select **Yes** at the pop-up menu to return to the office map.
   • Keep **Louise Parlet** as your patient and continue to the next exercise.

Exercise 4

 Online Activity—Completing an Insurance Claim for a Patient with Blue Cross/Blue Shield as Secondary Coverage

 30 minutes

   • Click on **Billing and Coding**.
   • Click on **Charts** and review forms and sections of the chart as needed to complete the following questions.

 • Refer to the Step-by-Step Claims Completion Guidelines for Blue Cross/Blue Shield in the textbook (Chapter 7).

1. Using the Patient Information Form, complete the appropriate box(es) in Block 1 and enter the patient's insurance ID number in Block 1a of the CMS-1500 claim form below. Continue completing the form through Block 13 (*Note:* Because this patient has an additional insurance policy, Blocks 9 through 9d will need to be completed.)

[CMS-1500 Health Insurance Claim Form]

2. Using the information on the patient's Encounter Form, complete Blocks 14 through 20 on the CMS-1500 claim form below. (*Note:* Dr. Hayler's NPI is 0002223334.)

14. DATE OF CURRENT ILLNESS (First symptom) OR INJURY (Accident) OR PREGNANCY(LMP) MM DD YY		15. IF PATIENT HAS HAD SAME OR SIMILAR ILLNESS GIVE FIRST DATE MM DD YY	16. DATES PATIENT UNABLE TO WORK IN CURRENT OCCUPATION MM DD YY MM DD YY FROM TO
17. NAME OF REFERRING PROVIDER OR OTHER SOURCE	17a. 17b. NPI		18. HOSPITALIZATION DATES RELATED TO CURRENT SERVICES MM DD YY MM DD YY FROM TO
19. RESERVED FOR LOCAL USE			20. OUTSIDE LAB? ☐ YES ☐ NO $ CHARGES

3. Using the information on the patient's Encounter Form and the diagnosis code information you prepared in Lesson 5, enter the appropriate diagnosis codes in Block 21 on the CMS-1500 claim form below.

21. DIAGNOSIS OR NATURE OF ILLNESS OR INJURY (Relate Items 1, 2, 3 or 4 to Item 24E by Line)		22. MEDICAID RESUBMISSION CODE ORIGINAL REF. NO.
1. ____.____	3. ____.____	
2. ____.____	4. ____.____	23. PRIOR AUTHORIZATION NUMBER

4. Using the information on the Encounter Form, the procedure code information that you prepared in Lesson 6, and the clinic's Fee Schedule, complete Blocks 24A through 24J on the CMS-1500 claim form below for each service/procedure provided.

24. A DATE(S) OF SERVICE From MM DD YY To MM DD YY	B PLACE OF SERVICE	C EMG	D. PROCEDURES, SERVICES, OR SUPPLIES (Explain Unusual Circumstances) CPT/HCPCS	MODIFIER	E DIAGNOSIS POINTER	F $ CHARGES	G DAYS OR UNITS	H EPSDT Family Plan	I ID. QUAL	J RENDERING PROVIDER ID. #	
1									NPI		
2									NPI		
3									NPI		
4									NPI		
5									NPI		
6									NPI		

PHYSICIAN OR SUPPLIER INFORMATION

Based on your completion of the claim form, answer the following questions related to specific fields that insurance carriers frequently report as problematic areas.

5. In Block 4, the policy holder's name should be entered as which of the following?
   a. LOUISE PARLET
   b. Parlet Louise
   c. PARLET SCOTT
   d. SAME

6. Was it necessary to complete Blocks 9 through 9d?
   a. No, the patient did not have an additional insurance policy.
   b. Yes, the patient had an additional insurance policy.

7. Block 14 reads, "ILLNESS (First Symptom) OR INJURY (Accident) OR PREGNANCY (LMP)." Does this block need to be completed for Ms. Parlet's claim?
   a. Yes
   b. No, this is not applicable to this case because there was no accident.

8. If it is necessary to enter the information in Block 14, where can you find the correct information to complete it?
a. On the Encounter Form
b. On the Patient Information Form
c. In the Progress Note
d. In the Diagnostic Tests section of the chart
e. By asking the patient directly

- Click **Close Chart** to return to the Billing and Coding area.
- Click the exit arrow.
- Click **Return to Map** and select **Yes** at the pop-up menu to return to the office map.

Exercise 5

 Online Activity—Completing a CMS-1500 Claim Form for a Patient with Private Insurance

 30 minutes

- Select **John R. Simmons** from the patient list.
- Click on **Billing and Coding**.
- Click on **Charts**.

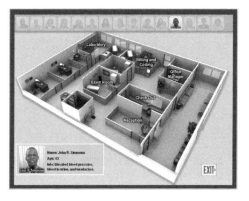

1. Complete a CMS-1500 claim form for John R. Simmons below.

• Click **Close Chart** to return to the Billing and Coding area.
• Click the exit arrow.
• Click **Exit the Program** or, if continuing to a new lesson, click **Return to Map** and then click **Yes** on the pop-up menu.

LESSON 12

Medicare

 Reading Assignment: Chapter 12—Medicare

Patients: Wilson Metcalf, Jean Deere, Hu Huang

Rooms: Reception, Check Out, Billing and Coding

Objectives:

- Understand essential points of the Medicare program.
- Identify the Medicare beneficiary and determine eligibility.
- Extract important patient information from a Medicare ID card.
- Identify the various Medicare combination coverages.
- Identify the benefits provided to Medicare beneficiaries.
- Identify patient cost-sharing responsibilities under Medicare.
- Differentiate between Part A and Part B benefits.
- Complete Medicare claim forms.
- Identify the benefits for a participating versus a nonparticipating physician.

Exercise 1

 Online Activity—Identifying the Medicare Beneficiary

15 minutes

- Sign in to Mountain View Clinic.
- Select **Wilson Metcalf** from the patient list.
- Click on **Reception**.
- Click on **Policy** to open the office Policy Manual.

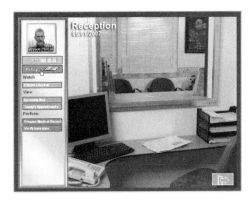

157

Answer the following questions, using Mountain View Clinic's Policy Manual and your knowledge of the Medicare program. Refer to Chapter 12 in your textbook for additional help.

1. Medicare is a federal health insurance program for which categories of people? Select all that apply.

_____ People 65 years of age or older who are on Social Security

_____ People 65 years of age or older who are retired from the railroad or civil service

_____ People 62 years of age or older who are on Social Security

_____ Disabled individuals who are eligible for Social Security disability benefits and disabled workers of any age

_____ Disabled individuals who are eligible for Social Security disability benefits but not disabled workers of any age

_____ Kidney donors

_____ Children and adults who have end-stage renal disease and require a kidney transplant

_____ Disabled widows of workers who are fully or currently insured through the federal government and whose husbands qualified for benefits under this program

2. Medicare is composed of four parts (A, B, C, and D). Office visits provided by physicians at Mountain View Clinic would be billed to which of these parts?
   a. Part A
   b. Part B
   c. Part C
   d. Part D

3. Which part of Medicare provides seniors and people living with disabilities with a prescription drug benefit?
   a. Part A
   b. Part B
   c. Part C
   d. Part D

4. The health insurance professional should know that Medicare is administered by the:
   a. Social Security Administration (SSA) office.
   b. Centers for Medicare and Medicaid Services (CMS).
   c. Office of the Aging.
   d. Department of Health and Human Services.

→ • Click **Close Manual** to return to the Reception area.
   • Remain in the Reception area with **Wilson Metcalf** as your patient and continue to the next exercise.

Exercise 2

Online Activity—Determining Medicare Eligibility

 15 minutes

- Under the Watch heading, click on **Patient Check-In** and watch the video.

 • You may refer to Chapter 12 in your textbook as needed to answer the following questions.

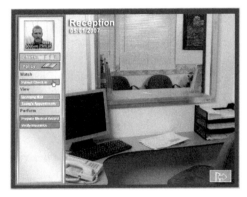

1. How did Kristin know that Mr. Metcalf was eligible for Medicare benefits?
   a. Kristin asked Mr. Metcalf whether his insurance had changed since his last visit.
   b. Kristin looked at his patient registration form.
   c. Kristin thought Mr. Metcalf looked like he was over 65.
   d. Kristin remembered that Mr. Metcalf had Medicare from his previous visit.

2. Mr. Metcalf stated that he is now covered under Medicare. When was he eligible for Medicare benefits?
   a. The first day of the year in which he turned 65.
   b. The first day of the month in which he turned 65.
   c. The day that he turned 65.
   d. The day that he applied for Social Security benefits.

3. When Kristin asked Mr. Metcalf for his Medicare card, he asked her what the card looked like. Kristin described the card by saying which of the following?
   a. It says Medicare across the top of it.
   b. It has your name on it.
   c. It has a picture of an eagle on it.
   d. It is printed in red, white, and blue.

4. Which of the following information is shown on the front of an authentic Medicare card? Select all that apply. (**Hint:** See Mr. Metcalf's Medicare card and your textbook for help.)

   _____ Name of beneficiary

   _____ Beneficiary's address and phone number

   _____ Medicare claim number

   _____ Beneficiary's sex

   _____ Beneficiary's telephone number

   _____ Date(s) beneficiary became eligible for Parts A and/or B

   _____ Medicare's toll-free phone number

   _____ Signature of beneficiary

5. Mr. Metcalf's Medicare number is 000456782A. What does the patient status letter "A" stand for at the end of the number?
   a. Nothing. All Medicare numbers end in A.
   b. It indicates that he is a returned wage earner.
   c. It indicates that he is a widower.
   d. It indicates that he is eligible for Part A benefits.

6. If Mr. Metcalf's Medicare number began with the patient status letter "A," it would indicate:
   a. that Mr. Metcalf is eligible for Part A benefits.
   b. that Mr. Metcalf is a railroad retiree.
   c. that Mr. Metcalf is a retired coal miner.
   d. none of the above; the patient status letter never precedes the Medicare number.

- Click the **X** to close the video.
- Click the exit arrow.
- Click **Return to Map** and select **Yes** at the pop-up menu to return to the office map.

Exercise 3

 Online Activity—Patient with Medicare Combination Coverage

 15 minutes

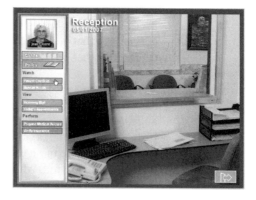

- Select **Jean Deere** from the patient list.
- Click on **Reception**.
- Under the Watch heading, click on **Patient Check-In** and watch the video.
- Click the **X** to close the video.
- Click on **Charts**.
 - Refer to Chapter 12 in your textbook as needed to answer the following questions.

1. The receptionist at Mountain View Clinic states that she will need to verify Ms. Deere's Patient Information Form. Upon review of the form and Ms. Deere's insurance cards, the receptionist will confirm that Ms. Deere has coverage through:
   a. Medicare only.
   b. Medicare/Medicaid (Oasis Health Care).
   c. Medicare and a Medicare Supplemental Insurance (Oasis Health Care).
   d. Medicare and a Medicare Advantage Plan (Oasis Health Care).

2. Ms. Deere's Medigap Insurance will cover:
   a. physician services.
   b. hospital services.
   c. pharmacy charges.
   d. health care expenses not covered by Medicare (deductibles and coinsurance).

3. Indicate whether each of the following statements is true or false.

    a. _____ Ms. Deere's insurance coverage under Oasis Health Care would be considered a Medicare Secondary Payer.

    b. _____ If Ms. Deere had simultaneous insurance coverage with Medicare and Medicaid, it would be referred to as Medi-Medi.

    c. _____ If Ms. Deere chose to receive Medicare benefits through a managed care plan rather than through traditional Medicare, she would have the same coverage, same premiums, and same coinsurance.

- Click **Close Chart** to return to the Reception area.
- Click the exit arrow.
- Click **Return to Map** and select **Yes** at the pop-up menu to return to the office map.

Exercise 4

Online Activity—Identifying the Benefits Provided to Medicare Beneficiaries

20 minutes

- Select **Hu Huang** from the patient list.
- Click on **Check Out**.
- Click on **Charts**.
- Click on the **Patient Information** tab and select **2-Insurance Cards**.

1. What type(s) of Medicare coverage is Mr. Huang entitled to?

2. If Mr. Huang needed to be admitted to the hospital as an inpatient, Medicare Part A would provide benefits to him as a "bed patient" for up to _____ hospital days for each benefit period.

3. As a Medicare beneficiary with Part B benefits, Mr. Huang will have to pay how much for all covered services provided at Mountain View Clinic?
   a. Nothing, Medicare will pay for all covered services.
   b. He will pay a yearly deductible only.
   c. He will pay a 20% deductible only.
   d. He will pay a yearly deductible and a 20% copayment.

4. For each service listed below, identify whether Medicare Part A or Part B would provide coverage.

   Type of Service   **Medicare Coverage**

   _____ Inpatient hospital care   a. Medicare Part A

   _____ Care in a skilled nursing facility   b. Medicare Part B

   _____ Ambulance transport

   _____ Diagnostic tests/x-rays

   _____ Emergency Department services

   _____ Physician services

   _____ Hospice

   _____ Home health care

   _____ Ambulatory care services

   _____ Blood products

5. Indicate whether each of the following statements regarding coverage of services is true or false.

   a. _____ Cosmetic surgery is considered a noncovered service.

   b. _____ The physician is not allowed to bill for a noncovered service.

   c. _____ Coverage requirements under Medicare state that for a service to be covered, it must be considered medically necessary.

6. How would the health insurance professional determine whether the test that the physician is ordering for Mr. Huang is considered medically necessary?

7. If the health insurance professional determines that the test the physician is ordering for Mr. Huang is not considered medically necessary, what action should be taken?

8. Mountain View Clinic has signed a participating physician agreement, which means that the clinic will accept payment from Medicare (_____% of the approved charge), plus payment from the patient (_____% of the approved charge).

9. If Mountain View Clinic were not participating with Medicare, the physician would receive only _____% of the Medicare-approved amount.

10. The nonparticipating physician may only bill Medicare beneficiaries a percentage of the Medicare-approved amount, as specified through legislation, known as the

_____ charge.

11. What is the most important reason for the health insurance professional to be able to answer Medicare patients' questions about their cost-sharing responsibilities accurately?
    a. It is not important; the primary job of the health insurance professional is to complete CMS-1500 claim forms.
    b. It will help to avoid Medicare claim denial.
    c. It will help to ensure timely filing of Medicare claims.
    d. The Medicare program is confusing, and older adults will need assistance in understanding the program.

➡ • Click **Close Chart** to return to the Check out area.
  • Click the exit arrow.
  • Click **Return to Map** and select **Yes** at the pop-up menu to return to the office map.
  • Keep Hu Huang as your patient and continue to the next exercise.

Exercise 5

 Online Activity—Completing a Medicare Claim

 40 minutes

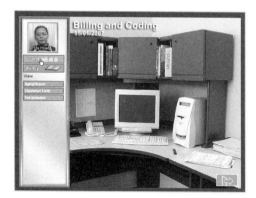

- Click on **Billing and Coding**.
- Click on **Charts**.

- For help with completion of the CMS-1500 form, refer to Chapters 7 and 12 of the textbook.
- For reference to diagnosis and procedure codes that were previously assigned, refer to Lessons 5 and 6.

1. Using the information in Hu Huang's medical record, complete the following CMS-1500 claim form for a Medicare claim.

1500

HEALTH INSURANCE CLAIM FORM

APPROVED BY NATIONAL UNIFORM CLAIM COMMITTEE 08/05

CARRIER

| | PICA | | | | | | | | | | PICA | |

| 1. MEDICARE | MEDICAID | TRICARE CHAMPUS | CHAMPVA | GROUP HEALTH PLAN | FECA BLK LUNG | OTHER | 1a. INSURED'S I.D. NUMBER | (For Program in Item 1) |
| (Medicare #) | (Medicaid #) | (Sponsor's SSN) | (Member ID#) | (SSN or ID) | (SSN) | (ID) | | |

2. PATIENT'S NAME (Last Name, First Name, Middle Initial)

3. PATIENT'S BIRTH DATE MM | DD | YY   SEX   M   F

4. INSURED'S NAME (Last Name, First Name, Middle Initial)

5. PATIENT'S ADDRESS (No., Street)

6. PATIENT RELATIONSHIP TO INSURED   Self   Spouse   Child   Other

7. INSURED'S ADDRESS (No., Street)

CITY   STATE

8. PATIENT STATUS   Single   Married   Other

CITY   STATE

ZIP CODE   TELEPHONE (Include Area Code) ( )

Employed   Full-Time Student   Part-Time Student

ZIP CODE   TELEPHONE (Include Area Code) ( )

9. OTHER INSURED'S NAME (Last Name, First Name, Middle Initial)

10. IS PATIENT'S CONDITION RELATED TO:

11. INSURED'S POLICY GROUP OR FECA NUMBER

a. OTHER INSURED'S POLICY OR GROUP NUMBER

a. EMPLOYMENT? (Current or Previous)   YES   NO

a. INSURED'S DATE OF BIRTH MM | DD | YY   SEX   M   F

b. OTHER INSURED'S DATE OF BIRTH MM | DD | YY   SEX   M   F

b. AUTO ACCIDENT?   YES   NO   PLACE (State)

b. EMPLOYER'S NAME OR SCHOOL NAME

c. EMPLOYER'S NAME OR SCHOOL NAME

c. OTHER ACCIDENT?   YES   NO

c. INSURANCE PLAN NAME OR PROGRAM NAME

d. INSURANCE PLAN NAME OR PROGRAM NAME

10d. RESERVED FOR LOCAL USE

d. IS THERE ANOTHER HEALTH BENEFIT PLAN?   YES   NO   *If yes*, return to and complete item 9 a-d.

READ BACK OF FORM BEFORE COMPLETING & SIGNING THIS FORM.
12. PATIENT'S OR AUTHORIZED PERSON'S SIGNATURE. I authorize the release of any medical or other information necessary to process this claim. I also request payment of government benefits either to myself or to the party who accepts assignment below.

SIGNED _____   DATE _____

13. INSURED'S OR AUTHORIZED PERSON'S SIGNATURE. I authorize payment of medical benefits to the undersigned physician or supplier for services described below.

SIGNED _____

14. DATE OF CURRENT: MM | DD | YY   ILLNESS (First symptom) OR INJURY (Accident) OR PREGNANCY(LMP)

15. IF PATIENT HAS HAD SAME OR SIMILAR ILLNESS GIVE FIRST DATE MM | DD | YY

16. DATES PATIENT UNABLE TO WORK IN CURRENT OCCUPATION MM | DD | YY FROM   TO   MM | DD | YY

17. NAME OF REFERRING PROVIDER OR OTHER SOURCE

17a.
17b. NPI

18. HOSPITALIZATION DATES RELATED TO CURRENT SERVICES MM | DD | YY FROM   TO   MM | DD | YY

19. RESERVED FOR LOCAL USE

20. OUTSIDE LAB?   YES   NO $ CHARGES

21. DIAGNOSIS OR NATURE OF ILLNESS OR INJURY (Relate Items 1, 2, 3 or 4 to Item 24E by Line)

1. _____   3. _____
2. _____   4. _____

22. MEDICAID RESUBMISSION CODE   ORIGINAL REF. NO.

23. PRIOR AUTHORIZATION NUMBER

24. A. DATE(S) OF SERVICE From MM DD YY To MM DD YY	B. PLACE OF SERVICE	C. EMG	D. PROCEDURES, SERVICES, OR SUPPLIES (Explain Unusual Circumstances) CPT/HCPCS	MODIFIER	E. DIAGNOSIS POINTER	F. $ CHARGES	G. DAYS OR UNITS	H. EPSDT Family Plan	I. ID QUAL	J. RENDERING PROVIDER ID. #
1										NPI
2										NPI
3										NPI
4										NPI
5										NPI
6										NPI

25. FEDERAL TAX I.D. NUMBER   SSN   EIN

26. PATIENT'S ACCOUNT NO.

27. ACCEPT ASSIGNMENT? (For govt. claims, see back)   YES   NO

28. TOTAL CHARGE $

29. AMOUNT PAID $

30. BALANCE DUE $

31. SIGNATURE OF PHYSICIAN OR SUPPLIER INCLUDING DEGREES OR CREDENTIALS (I certify that the statements on the reverse apply to this bill and are made a part thereof.)

SIGNED _____   DATE _____

32. SERVICE FACILITY LOCATION INFORMATION

a.   b.

33. BILLING PROVIDER INFO & PH # ( )

a.   b.

PATIENT AND INSURED INFORMATION   PHYSICIAN OR SUPPLIER INFORMATION

NUCC Instruction Manual available at: www.nucc.org

APPROVED OMB-0938-0999 FORM CMS-1500 (08/05)

- Click **Close Chart** to return to the Billing and Coding area.
- Click the exit arrow.
- Click **Return to Map** and select **Yes** at the pop-up menu to return to the office map.
- Select **Jean Deere** from the patient list.
- Click on **Billing and Coding**.
- Click on **Charts**.

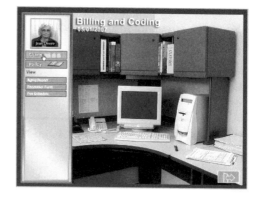

2. Using the information in Jean Deere's medical record, complete the following CMS-1500 claim form for a Medicare claim.

• Click **Close Chart** to return to the Billing & Coding area.
 • Click the exit arrow.
 • Click **Exit the Program** or, if continuing to a new lesson, click **Return to Map** and then click **Yes** on the pop-up menu.

13

Medicaid and Other State Programs

👓 **Reading Assignment:** Chapter 13—Medicaid and Other State Programs

Patients: Rhea Davison, Wilson Metcalf

Rooms: Check Out, Billing and Coding

Objectives:

- Demonstrate an understanding of the Medicaid program.
- Determine Medicaid eligibility.
- Identify the different types of Medicaid programs.
- Understand Medicaid coverage.
- Identify Medicaid basic benefit services.
- Understand Medicaid payment policies.
- Complete a Medicaid claim.

Exercise 1

 Online Activity—Understanding the Medicaid Program

 20 minutes

- Sign in to Mountain View Clinic.
- Select **Rhea Davison** from the patient list.
- Click on **Check Out**.
- Click on **Policy** to open the office Policy Manual.

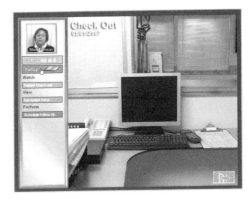

Answer the following questions, using Mountain View Clinic's Policy Manual and your knowledge of the Medicaid program based on information in the textbook.

1. Medicaid is a:
   a. commercial health insurance plan.
   b. managed care plan.
   c. federal and state health insurance program.
   d. federal and state medical assistance program.

2. The Medicaid program covers patients:
   a. whose employers have selected the program as their insurance plan.
   b. who are over the age of 65 years old.
   c. who are needy and whose incomes are low.
   d. who have end-stage renal disease (ESRD).

3. Indicate whether each of the following statements is true or false.

   a. _____ Mountain View Clinic participates with the Medicaid program.

   b. _____ Based on federal and state guidelines, Mountain View Clinic must accept Medicaid patients.

   c. _____ Medicaid coverage and benefits vary widely from state to state.

   d. _____ Providers do not need to enroll to participate in the Medicaid program; they are automatically enrolled.

   e. _____ Time limits for filing Medicaid claims is the same for all states (90 days).

   f. _____ The CMS-1500 form is used for processing Medicaid claims in all states.

   g. _____ Medicaid Fraud Control Units investigate all alleged cases of fraud in all states.

4. If the physicians at Mountain View Clinic decide to limit the number of Medicaid patients they see and therefore no longer accept new Medicaid patients, what procedure should the medical receptionist follow if a Medicaid patient insists on being seen anyway?
   a. Refuse to schedule any appointments for the patient.
   b. Inform the patient that the practice does not accept Medicaid patients and offer to schedule the appointment if the patient agrees to pay for the service.

→ • Remain in the Check Out area with **Rhea Davison** as your patient and continue to the next exercise.

Exercise 2

Online Activity—Understanding Medicaid Eligibility and the Different Types of Medicaid Programs

15 minutes

1. A Medicaid identification card is usually issued:
   a. weekly.
   b. monthly.
   c. yearly.
   d. once a lifetime.

2. To determine Medicaid eligibility, the patient's Medicaid ID card should be verified at every visit or at least:
   a. once a week.
   b. once a month.
   c. once every 6 months.
   d. once a year.

3. When verifying eligibility of Medicaid coverage with the ID card, it is important to confirm:
   a. the eligibility period.
   b. the policy holder's name.
   c. the patient's PCP.
   d. the need for preauthorization or precertification.

4. There are three aid programs for eligible Medicare patients with low incomes who have difficulty paying Medicare premiums, copayments, and deductibles. Match each program with its description of eligibility.

Low-Income Medicare Program	Description of Eligibility
_____ Qualified Medicare Beneficiary Program	a. Older adults whose income is no more than 20% above the federal poverty level.
_____ Specialized Low-Income Medicare Beneficiary Program	b. Medicare beneficiaries who are aged and disabled and have annual incomes below the federal poverty level
_____ Qualifying Individual Program	c. Individuals whose income is at least 135% but less than 175% of the federal poverty level.

 • Remain in the Check Out area with **Rhea Davison** as your patient and continue to the next exercise.

Exercise 3

Online Activity—Identifying Medicaid Coverage

 15 minutes

- Under the Watch heading, click on **Patient Check-Out** and watch the video.

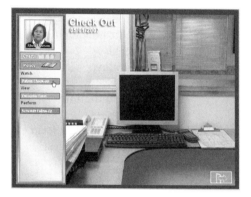

1. Identify the type of health insurance Rhea Davison has.
   a. Commercial insurance
   b. Managed care
   c. Medicaid
   d. None

2. How has Ms. Davison been paying for her medical services?
   a. By credit card
   b. Through her employer
   c. Through a payment plan set up by the clinic
   d. By providing child care for the physician's children

3. In the video, what does the medical assistant suggest to Ms. Davison to help her with paying for ongoing care?
   a. She offers to give Ms. Davison a discount.
   b. She offers to give Ms. Davison information on government-sponsored programs.
   c. She encourages her to enroll in Medicare.
   d. She encourages her to obtain a credit card so services can be charged.

4. If Ms. Davison is accepted for Medicaid at her next visit, she will bring a form or card to the office. Does this indicate proof of eligibility? Why or why not?

5. Title XIX of the Social Security Act requires that certain basic services be offered to certain eligible groups. Which of the following services/procedures would qualify as Medicaid basic benefits and be available to Ms. Davison? Select all that apply. (***Hint:*** Use your textbook for assistance, if needed.)

_____ Physician services

_____ Laboratory and x-ray services

_____ Plastic surgery (face lifts, tummy tucks, liposuction)

_____ Home health care

_____ Nursing facility services

_____ Dental services (x-rays, cleaning, fillings)

_____ Inpatient/outpatient hospital services

_____ Prescription and over-the-counter drugs

 • Click the **X** on the video screen to close the video.
 • Click the exit arrow.
 • Click **Return to Map** and select **Yes** at the pop-up menu to return to the office map.
 • Keep **Rhea Davison** as your patient and continue to the next exercise.

Exercise 4

 Online Activity—Medicaid Payment Policies

15 minutes

In this exercise, we will assume that Rhea Davison has met the criteria to receive Medicaid benefits and is eligible for coverage on this date of service.

 • Click on **Billing and Coding**.
 • Click on the **Encounter Form** clipboard.

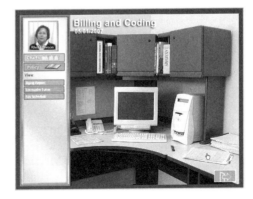

1. According to the Encounter Form, Ms. Davison received the following services during today's visit. Which of these procedures or services would qualify as "medically necessary" and be payable under Medicaid? Select all that apply.

_____ Established patient visit, level IV

_____ Blood glucose test

_____ Pap smear

_____ UA dipstick

_____ Hemoccult

2. Many times, prior approval is necessary for Medicaid coverage of certain services, except in a true emergency. Which of the following products or services would require prior approval to ensure payment by Medicaid? Select all that apply.

_____ Hearing aids

_____ Durable medical equipment

_____ Outpatient office visits

_____ Laboratory procedures

_____ Medications

_____ Surgical procedures

_____ Allergy care

_____ Some vision care

3. If a service requires prior approval, and it is not approved, how would the office be paid for the services provided?

4. Indicate whether the each of the following statements is true or false.

a. _____ Under Medicaid regulations, Ms. Davison will never have a share of cost as long as she is eligible for Medicaid benefits.

b. _____ Medicaid payments will be made directly to the patient.

c. _____ Providers participating in the Medicaid program must accept Medicaid-approved amounts as payment in full.

d. _____ Medicaid is considered the payer of last resort.

5. Medicaid reimbursements are calculated:
   a. by the provider.
   b. by the county health department.
   c. by the state health department.
   d. by the federal health department.

 • Click **Finish** to return to the Check Out area.
   • Click the exit arrow.
   • Click **Return to Map** and select **Yes** at the pop-up menu to return to the office map.

Exercise 5

 Online Activity—Completing a Medicaid Claim for the Medicare/Medicaid Patient

 30 minutes

   • Select **Wilson Metcalf** from the patient list.
   • Click on **Billing and Coding**.
   • Click on **Charts**.

1. According to the Patient Information section of the chart, Mr. Metcalf now has Medicare. Let's also assume that because of Mr. Metcalf's income level, which is below the federal poverty level, he qualifies for Medicaid, which will provide limited coverage, including:
   a. Medicare premiums.
   b. Medicare deductibles.
   c. Medicare coinsurance amounts.
   d. all of the above.

2. If Mr. Metcalf has both Medicare and Medicaid coverage, a claim should be sent first to:
   a. Medicaid.
   b. Medicare.

3. If Mr. Metcalf's claim is not submitted to Medicaid within the time limit set by the state:
   a. the provider may bill the patient.
   b. the provider may not bill the patient.

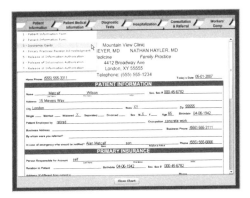 • Click on the **Patient Information** tab and select **3-Insurance Cards**.

4. Using the guidelines in the textbook (Chapter 7) complete the Patient/Insured section of the CMS-1500 form below for Mr. Metcalf. (***Remember:*** He is now dual eligible. Report his Medicaid identification number as MCDxxxxxxxxx.)

1500

HEALTH INSURANCE CLAIM FORM

APPROVED BY NATIONAL UNIFORM CLAIM COMMITTEE 08/05

```
PICA                                                                                    PICA

1 MEDICARE     MEDICAID      TRICARE        CHAMPVA      GROUP        FECA        OTHER   1a INSURED'S I.D. NUMBER              (For Program in item 1)
                             CHAMPUS                     HEALTH PLAN  BLK LUNG
  (Medicare #)  (Medicaid #) (Sponsor's SSN) (Member ID#) (SSN or ID) (SSN)        (ID)

2 PATIENT'S NAME (Last Name, First Name, Middle Initial)   3 PATIENT'S BIRTH DATE    SEX    4 INSURED'S NAME (Last Name, First Name, Middle Initial)
                                                            MM   DD   YY
                                                                            M     F

5 PATIENT'S ADDRESS (No., Street)                          6 PATIENT RELATIONSHIP TO INSURED   7 INSURED'S ADDRESS (No., Street)
                                                            Self   Spouse   Child   Other

CITY                                              STATE    8 PATIENT STATUS                    CITY                                      STATE
                                                            Single   Married   Other

ZIP CODE          TELEPHONE (Include Area Code)                                                ZIP CODE          TELEPHONE (Include Area Code)
                  (    )                                   Employed   Full-Time   Part-Time                     (    )
                                                                      Student     Student

9 OTHER INSURED'S NAME (Last Name, First Name, Middle Initial)  10 IS PATIENT'S CONDITION RELATED TO:   11 INSURED'S POLICY GROUP OR FECA NUMBER

a OTHER INSURED'S POLICY OR GROUP NUMBER                    a EMPLOYMENT? (Current or Previous)  a INSURED'S DATE OF BIRTH              SEX
                                                              YES       NO                           MM   DD   YY          M       F

b OTHER INSURED'S DATE OF BIRTH          SEX                b AUTO ACCIDENT?         PLACE (State)   b EMPLOYER'S NAME OR SCHOOL NAME
  MM   DD   YY                  M     F                       YES       NO

c EMPLOYER'S NAME OR SCHOOL NAME                            c OTHER ACCIDENT?                      c INSURANCE PLAN NAME OR PROGRAM NAME
                                                             YES       NO

d INSURANCE PLAN NAME OR PROGRAM NAME                       10d RESERVED FOR LOCAL USE           d IS THERE ANOTHER HEALTH BENEFIT PLAN?
                                                                                                    YES       NO    If yes, return to and complete item 9 a-d

READ BACK OF FORM BEFORE COMPLETING & SIGNING THIS FORM.
12 PATIENT'S OR AUTHORIZED PERSON'S SIGNATURE. I authorize the release of any medical or other information necessary   13 INSURED'S OR AUTHORIZED PERSON'S SIGNATURE. I authorize
to process this claim. I also request payment of government benefits either to myself or to the party who accepts assignment   payment of medical benefits to the undersigned physician or supplier for
below                                                                                                   services described below

SIGNED_____   DATE_____          SIGNED_____
```

CARRIER — PATIENT AND INSURED INFORMATION

 • Click **Close Chart** to return to the Billing and Coding area.
• Click the exit arrow.
• Click **Exit the Program** or, if continuing to a new lesson, click **Return to Map** and then click **Yes** on the pop-up menu.

LESSON 14

TRICARE and CHAMPVA

 Reading Assignment: Chapter 14—TRICARE and CHAMPVA

Patients: Rhea Davison, Jesus Santo

Room: Check Out

Objectives:

- Identify the TRICARE beneficiary and determine eligibility.
- Identify various TRICARE programs and payment types.
- Identify TRICARE claim submission and reimbursement policies.
- Identify the CHAMPVA beneficiary and determine eligibility.
- Determine CHAMPVA benefits, preauthorization, and reimbursement policies.
- Complete a claim for a TRICARE and for a CHAMPVA patient.

Exercise 1

 Online Activity—The TRICARE Patient

 30 minutes

1. TRICARE is a health care program that provides coverage to:
   a. active-duty or retired members of the military services and their families.
   b. individuals over 65 years old.
   c. parents of active-duty military service members.
   d. dependents of veterans with service-related disabilities.

→ • Sign in to Mountain View Clinic.
- Select **Rhea Davison** from the patient list.
- Click on **Check Out**.
- Click on **Charts**.
- Click on the **Patient Medical Information** tab and select **1-Patient Information Form**.

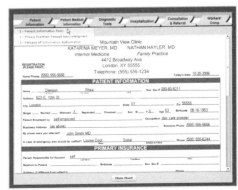

177

2. What type of insurance coverage does Ms. Davison have, if any?
   a. She has no insurance coverage; she is a "self-pay" patient.
   b. She has TRICARE.
   c. She has CHAMPUS.
   d. She has CHAMPVA.

3. Ms. Davison has married, resulting in a change in her insurance coverage. Complete the primary insurance section of Ms. Davison's Patient Information Form using the following information:

   - Sponsor: Arthur T. Bentler (spouse)
   - SSN: 000123456
   - Birth date: 03/10/1959
   - Employer: U.S. Army
   - Occupation: Reservist
   - Address: Use patient's address for the sponsor as well
   - *Note:* Rhea Davison now goes by the married name of Rhea Davison-Bentler).

PRIMARY INSURANCE

Person Responsible for Account _____
                                   Last Name   First Name   Initial

Relation to Patient _____ Birthdate _____ Soc. Sec.# _____

Address (if different from patient's) _____ Phone _____

City _____ State _____ Zip _____

Person Responsible Employed by _____ Occupation _____

Business Address _____ Business Phone _____

Insurance Company _____

Contract # _____ Group # _____ Subscriber # _____

Name of other dependents covered under this plan _____

4. Ms. Davison-Bentler is eligible for coverage under which of the following military programs?
   a. MHP
   b. TRICARE
   c. CHAMPVA
   d. DEERS

5. For which of the following programs, if any, is Ms. Davison-Bentler eligible? Select all that apply.

   _____ TRICARE Standard

   _____ TRICARE Extra

   _____ TRICARE Prime

   _____ CHAMPVA

   _____ TRICARE for Life

6. Who would be considered the sponsor for her coverage under this military program?
   a. The patient, Rhea Davison-Bentler
   b. Her husband, Arthur Bentler
   c. The U.S. Army Reserve
   d. The federal government

7. Immediately after her enrollment, Rhea Davison-Bentler's information is entered into the national computerized military database. What is the acronym for this database?
   a. MHS
   b. MTF
   c. DEERS
   d. TAMP

8. Which TRICARE program would Rhea Davison-Bentler be enrolled in if she does not pay an enrollment fee?
   a. TRICARE Standard
   b. TRICARE Extra
   c. TRICARE Prime
   d. TRICARE Standard Supplemental

9. Let's assume that Rhea Davison-Bentler enrolls in TRICARE Standard and that the Mountain View Clinic physicians are listed in the TRICARE Provider Directory. Under which TRICARE program would she essentially be receiving benefits?
   a. TRICARE Standard
   b. TRICARE Extra
   c. TRICARE Prime
   d. TRICARE for Life

10. If Rhea Davison-Bentler enrolls in TRICARE Standard and receives treatment from a physician at Mountain View Clinic who is not a participating physician with TRICARE, how much will the patient be responsible for?
    a. The entire fee charged by Mountain View Clinic.
    b. Only the TRICARE allowable charge.
    c. 15% above the TRICARE allowable charge.
    d. Only the cost share and deductible, if any.

11. The health insurance professional at Mountain View Clinic should be aware that the deadline for submitting claims to TRICARE is:
    a. 30 days from the date services were rendered.
    b. 90 days from the date services were rendered.
    c. 1 year from the date services were rendered.
    d. 2 years from the date services were rendered.

→ • Click **Close Chart** to return to the Check Out area.
  • Click the exit arrow.
  • Click **Return to Map** and select **Yes** at the pop-up menu to return to the office map.

Exercise 2

Online Activity—The CHAMPVA Patient

 25 minutes

1. CHAMPVA is:
   a. the same as TRICARE.
   b. for active-duty members of the military services and their families.
   c. for retired members of the military services and their dependents.
   d. for veterans with permanent service-related disabilities and their spouses, dependents, or survivors.

- Select **Jesus Santo** from the patient list.
- Click on **Reception**.
- Under the Watch heading, click on **Patient Check-In** and watch video.
- Click the **X** on the video screen to close the video.
- Click the exit arrow.
- Click **Return to Map** and select **Yes** at the pop-up menu to return to the office map.
- Click on **Check Out**.
- Under the Watch heading, click on **Patient Check-Out** and watch the video.
- Click the **X** on the video screen to close the video.
- Click the exit arrow.
- Click **Return to Map** and select **Yes** at the pop-up menu to return to the office map.
- Click on **Billing and Coding**.
- Click on **Charts**.

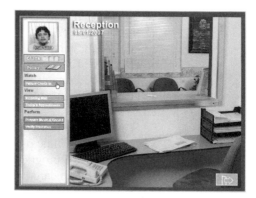

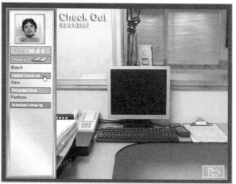

For this exercise, assume that while taking a detailed history of Mr. Santo, a member of the health care team discovers that the patient is the surviving spouse of Anita L. Santo, a veteran of Desert Storm who died from service-related injuries.

2. In this case, is Mr. Santo eligible to receive CHAMPVA health care benefits? Which of the following most accurately explains why or why not?
   a. No, only the dependent children of Ms. Santo would be eligible for coverage.
   b. No, Mr. Santo would be eligible for benefits under CHAMPUS.
   c. Yes, Mr. Santo is eligible for benefits under CHAMPVA since his wife served in the military.
   d. Yes, Mr. Santo is eligible for benefits under CHAMPVA since he is the surviving spouse of a person who died of service-related injuries.

3. Mr. Santo will no longer eligible for CHAMPVA health care benefits:
   a. if he remarries.
   b. if he becomes eligible for TRICARE.
   c. if he becomes eligible for Medicare.
   d. if any of the above situations occur.

4. Below, complete the primary insurance section of Mr. Santo's Patient Information Form using the following information:

   • Sponsor's name: Anita L. Santo (deceased)
   • SSN: 000121234
   • Date of birth: 12/06/1979
   • Relationship to patient: spouse
   • Address: Same as patient's

PRIMARY INSURANCE

Person Responsible for Account _____ Last Name _____ First Name _____ Initial

Relation to Patient _____ Birthdate _____ Soc. Sec.# _____

Address (if different from patient's) _____ Phone _____

City _____ State _____ Zip _____

Person Responsible Employed by _____ Occupation _____

Business Address _____ Business Phone _____

Insurance Company _____

Contract # _____ Group # _____ Subscriber # _____

Name of other dependents covered under this plan _____

5. The staff at Mountain View Clinic should confirm CHAMPVA eligibility by doing which of the following? Select all that apply.

   _____ Using the DEERS system

   _____ Using the IVR system

   _____ Making EDI requests through the EDI clearinghouse

   _____ Examining and copying the patient's CHAMPVA card

6. Indicate whether each of the following statements is true or false.

   a. _____ The physicians at Mountain View Clinic do not list CHAMPVA as an insurance that they participate with. Therefore they will not be able to treat Mr. Santos.

   b. _____ CHAMPVA will cover 75% of all health care services that Mr. Santo will receive.

7. CHAMPVA benefits include which of the following? Select all that apply.

_____ Prescription medication by mail

_____ Over-the-counter medications

_____ Dental care

_____ Eye care

8. Under CHAMPVA, preauthorization is required for:
   a. visits by specialists.
   b. diagnostic radiology services.
   c. mental health.
   d. laboratory services.

9. The CHAMPVA fee schedule is based on:
   a. the fee charged by the provider at Mountain View Clinic.
   b. the Medicare rate.
   c. 15% of the TRICARE fee schedule.
   d. the usual, reasonable, and customary rates.

10. CHAMPVA is always considered the secondary payer unless the services are also covered by:
    a. Medicaid.
    b. Medicare.
    c. any third-party payer.
    d. workers' compensation.

 • Click **Close Chart** to return to the Billing and Coding area.
• Click the exit arrow.
• Click **Exit the Program** or, if continuing to a new lesson, click **Return to Map** and then click **Yes** on the pop-up menu.

Exercise 3

 Online Activity—Completing Claims for TRICARE/CHAMPVA-Eligible Patients

 45 minutes

In this exercise, you will complete a TRICARE claim form for Rhea Davison-Bentler and a CHAMPVA claim for Jesus Santos, using the patient information from Exercises 1 and 2 of this lesson.

 For additional help, refer to Chapter 7 in your textbook, along with the Patient Information Forms you completed in Exercises 1 and 2 of this lesson.

1. Below, complete Blocks 1 through 33 for patient Rhea Davison-Bentler.

```
┌─────────┐
│  1500   │
└─────────┘
HEALTH INSURANCE CLAIM FORM
APPROVED BY NATIONAL UNIFORM CLAIM COMMITTEE 08/05
```

CARRIER

```
☐☐ PICA                                                                                                 PICA ☐☐

1  MEDICARE      MEDICAID      TRICARE       CHAMPVA      GROUP          FECA       OTHER    1a. INSURED'S I.D. NUMBER              (For Program in Item 1)
                               CHAMPUS                    HEALTH PLAN    BLK LUNG
   ☐(Medicare #) ☐(Medicaid #) ☐(Sponsor's SSN) ☐(Member ID#) ☐(SSN or ID) ☐(SSN) ☐(ID)

2  PATIENT'S NAME (Last Name, First Name, Middle Initial)      9  PATIENT'S BIRTH DATE      SEX      4  INSURED'S NAME (Last Name, First Name, Middle Initial)
                                                                 MM | DD | YY
                                                                            M☐  F☐

5  PATIENT'S ADDRESS (No., Street)                            6  PATIENT RELATIONSHIP TO INSURED   7  INSURED'S ADDRESS (No., Street)
                                                                Self☐ Spouse☐ Child☐ Other☐

CITY                                          STATE           8  PATIENT STATUS                    CITY                                    STATE
                                                                Single☐  Married☐  Other☐

ZIP CODE          TELEPHONE (Include Area Code)                                                  ZIP CODE        TELEPHONE (Include Area Code)
                  (   )                                       Employed☐ Full-Time☐ Part-Time☐                    (   )
                                                                         Student   Student

9  OTHER INSURED'S NAME (Last Name, First Name, Middle Initial)  10 IS PATIENT'S CONDITION RELATED TO  11 INSURED'S POLICY GROUP OR FECA NUMBER

a  OTHER INSURED'S POLICY OR GROUP NUMBER                      a  EMPLOYMENT? (Current or Previous)   a  INSURED'S DATE OF BIRTH          SEX
                                                                 ☐YES   ☐NO                             MM | DD | YY               M☐   F☐

b  OTHER INSURED'S DATE OF BIRTH      SEX                      b  AUTO ACCIDENT?     PLACE (State)    b  EMPLOYER'S NAME OR SCHOOL NAME
   MM | DD | YY          M☐   F☐                                 ☐YES   ☐NO

c  EMPLOYER'S NAME OR SCHOOL NAME                             c  OTHER ACCIDENT?                     c  INSURANCE PLAN NAME OR PROGRAM NAME
                                                                 ☐YES   ☐NO

d  INSURANCE PLAN NAME OR PROGRAM NAME                       10d RESERVED FOR LOCAL USE             d  IS THERE ANOTHER HEALTH BENEFIT PLAN?
                                                                                                      ☐YES  ☐NO   If yes, return to and complete item 9 a-d.

            READ BACK OF FORM BEFORE COMPLETING & SIGNING THIS FORM.              13 INSURED'S OR AUTHORIZED PERSON'S SIGNATURE I authorize
12 PATIENT'S OR AUTHORIZED PERSON'S SIGNATURE I authorize the release of any medical or other information necessary   payment of medical benefits to the undersigned physician or supplier for
   to process this claim. I also request payment of government benefits either to myself or to the party who accepts assignment   services described below.
   below.
   SIGNED_____     DATE_____            SIGNED_____
```

PATIENT AND INSURED INFORMATION

```
14 DATE OF CURRENT:  ◄ ILLNESS (First symptom) OR   15 IF PATIENT HAS HAD SAME OR SIMILAR ILLNESS   16 DATES PATIENT UNABLE TO WORK IN CURRENT OCCUPATION
   MM | DD | YY        INJURY (Accident) OR            GIVE FIRST DATE  MM | DD | YY                   MM | DD | YY            MM | DD | YY
                       PREGNANCY(LMP)                                                              FROM               TO

17 NAME OF REFERRING PROVIDER OR OTHER SOURCE      17a                                          18 HOSPITALIZATION DATES RELATED TO CURRENT SERVICES
                                                   17b NPI                                          MM | DD | YY            MM | DD | YY
                                                                                               FROM               TO

19 RESERVED FOR LOCAL USE                                                                      20 OUTSIDE LAB?          $ CHARGES
                                                                                                  ☐YES  ☐NO

21 DIAGNOSIS OR NATURE OF ILLNESS OR INJURY (Relate Items 1, 2, 3 or 4 to Item 24E by Line)    22 MEDICAID RESUBMISSION
                                                                                                  CODE          ORIGINAL REF. NO.
1 |___.___                    3 |___.___
                                                                                              23 PRIOR AUTHORIZATION NUMBER
2 |___.___                    4 |___.___

24 A  DATE(S) OF SERVICE        B      C   D PROCEDURES, SERVICES, OR SUPPLIES   E        F           G    H    I      J
      From        To        PLACE OF    EMG   (Explain Unusual Circumstances)  DIAGNOSIS  $ CHARGES  DAYS EPSDT ID    RENDERING
   MM DD YY   MM DD YY       SERVICE      CPT/HCPCS        MODIFIER            POINTER               OR   Family QUAL  PROVIDER ID. #
                                                                                                    UNITS Plan

1  |  |  |   |  |  |   |    |    |      |      |      |      |      |     |                           |    |         NPI

2  |  |  |   |  |  |   |    |    |      |      |      |      |      |     |                           |    |         NPI

3  |  |  |   |  |  |   |    |    |      |      |      |      |      |     |                           |    |         NPI

4  |  |  |   |  |  |   |    |    |      |      |      |      |      |     |                           |    |         NPI

5  |  |  |   |  |  |   |    |    |      |      |      |      |      |     |                           |    |         NPI

6  |  |  |   |  |  |   |    |    |      |      |      |      |      |     |                           |    |         NPI

25 FEDERAL TAX I.D. NUMBER    SSN EIN   26 PATIENT'S ACCOUNT NO.   27 ACCEPT ASSIGNMENT?   28 TOTAL CHARGE   29 AMOUNT PAID   30 BALANCE DUE
                              ☐                                      (For govt. claims, see back)
                                                                    ☐YES  ☐NO            $                $              $

31 SIGNATURE OF PHYSICIAN OR SUPPLIER    32 SERVICE FACILITY LOCATION INFORMATION   33 BILLING PROVIDER INFO & PH # (   )
   INCLUDING DEGREES OR CREDENTIALS
   (I certify that the statements on the reverse
   apply to this bill and are made a part thereof.)

SIGNED_____ DATE_____    a.           b.                               a.            b.
```

PHYSICIAN OR SUPPLIER INFORMATION

NUCC Instruction Manual available at: www.nucc.org   APPROVED OMB-0938-0999 FORM CMS-1500 (08/05)

2. Below, complete Blocks 1 through 33 for patient Jesus Santos.

1500

HEALTH INSURANCE CLAIM FORM

APPROVED BY NATIONAL UNIFORM CLAIM COMMITTEE 08/05

CARRIER

☐☐ PICA   PICA ☐☐☐

1. MEDICARE	MEDICAID	TRICARE CHAMPUS	CHAMPVA	GROUP HEALTH PLAN	FECA BLK LUNG	OTHER	1a. INSURED'S I.D. NUMBER (For Program in Item 1)
☐ (Medicare #)	☐ (Medicaid #)	☐ (Sponsor's SSN)	☐ (Member ID#)	☐ (SSN or ID)	☐ (SSN)	☐ (ID)	

2. PATIENT'S NAME (Last Name, First Name, Middle Initial)

3. PATIENT'S BIRTH DATE MM | DD | YY   SEX M☐ F☐

4. INSURED'S NAME (Last Name, First Name, Middle Initial)

5. PATIENT'S ADDRESS (No., Street)

6. PATIENT RELATIONSHIP TO INSURED
Self ☐ Spouse ☐ Child ☐ Other ☐

7. INSURED'S ADDRESS (No., Street)

CITY   STATE

8. PATIENT STATUS
Single ☐ Married ☐ Other ☐
Employed ☐ Full-Time Student ☐ Part-Time Student ☐

CITY   STATE

ZIP CODE   TELEPHONE (Include Area Code) (   )

ZIP CODE   TELEPHONE (Include Area Code) (   )

9. OTHER INSURED'S NAME (Last Name, First Name, Middle Initial)

10. IS PATIENT'S CONDITION RELATED TO:

11. INSURED'S POLICY GROUP OR FECA NUMBER

a. OTHER INSURED'S POLICY OR GROUP NUMBER

a. EMPLOYMENT? (Current or Previous) ☐ YES ☐ NO

a. INSURED'S DATE OF BIRTH MM | DD | YY   SEX M☐ F☐

b. OTHER INSURED'S DATE OF BIRTH MM | DD | YY   SEX M☐ F☐

b. AUTO ACCIDENT? PLACE (State) ☐ YES ☐ NO

b. EMPLOYER'S NAME OR SCHOOL NAME

c. EMPLOYER'S NAME OR SCHOOL NAME

c. OTHER ACCIDENT? ☐ YES ☐ NO

c. INSURANCE PLAN NAME OR PROGRAM NAME

d. INSURANCE PLAN NAME OR PROGRAM NAME

10d. RESERVED FOR LOCAL USE

d. IS THERE ANOTHER HEALTH BENEFIT PLAN?
☐ YES ☐ NO If yes, return to and complete item 9 a-d.

READ BACK OF FORM BEFORE COMPLETING & SIGNING THIS FORM.

12. PATIENT'S OR AUTHORIZED PERSON'S SIGNATURE I authorize the release of any medical or other information necessary to process this claim. I also request payment of government benefits either to myself or to the party who accepts assignment below.

SIGNED   DATE

13. INSURED'S OR AUTHORIZED PERSON'S SIGNATURE I authorize payment of medical benefits to the undersigned physician or supplier for services described below.

SIGNED

PATIENT AND INSURED INFORMATION

14. DATE OF CURRENT MM | DD | YY ILLNESS (First symptom) OR INJURY (Accident) OR PREGNANCY(LMP)

15. IF PATIENT HAS HAD SAME OR SIMILAR ILLNESS GIVE FIRST DATE MM | DD | YY

16. DATES PATIENT UNABLE TO WORK IN CURRENT OCCUPATION FROM MM | DD | YY   TO MM | DD | YY

17. NAME OF REFERRING PROVIDER OR OTHER SOURCE

17a.
17b. NPI

18. HOSPITALIZATION DATES RELATED TO CURRENT SERVICES FROM MM | DD | YY   TO MM | DD | YY

19. RESERVED FOR LOCAL USE

20. OUTSIDE LAB? ☐ YES ☐ NO $ CHARGES

21. DIAGNOSIS OR NATURE OF ILLNESS OR INJURY (Relate Items 1, 2, 3 or 4 to Item 24E by Line)
1.
2.
3.
4.

22. MEDICAID RESUBMISSION CODE   ORIGINAL REF. NO.

23. PRIOR AUTHORIZATION NUMBER

24. A. DATE(S) OF SERVICE From MM DD YY To MM DD YY	B. PLACE OF SERVICE	C. EMG	D. PROCEDURES, SERVICES, OR SUPPLIES (Explain Unusual Circumstances) CPT/HCPCS MODIFIER	E. DIAGNOSIS POINTER	F. $ CHARGES	G. DAYS OR UNITS	H. EPSDT Family Plan	I. ID QUAL	J. RENDERING PROVIDER ID. #
1									NPI
2									NPI
3									NPI
4									NPI
5									NPI
6									NPI

25. FEDERAL TAX I.D. NUMBER   SSN ☐ EIN ☐

26. PATIENT'S ACCOUNT NO.

27. ACCEPT ASSIGNMENT? (For govt. claims, see back) ☐ YES ☐ NO

28. TOTAL CHARGE $

29. AMOUNT PAID $

30. BALANCE DUE $

31. SIGNATURE OF PHYSICIAN OR SUPPLIER INCLUDING DEGREES OR CREDENTIALS (I certify that the statements on the reverse apply to this bill and are made a part thereof.)

SIGNED   DATE

32. SERVICE FACILITY LOCATION INFORMATION

a.   b.

33. BILLING PROVIDER INFO & PH # (   )

a.   b.

PHYSICIAN OR SUPPLIER INFORMATION

NUCC Instruction Manual available at: www.nucc.org

APPROVED OMB-0938-0999 FORM CMS-1500 (08/05)

LESSON 15

Workers' Compensation

Reading Assignment: Chapter 15—Workers' Compensation

Patient: Janet Jones

Rooms: Reception, Check Out

Objectives:

- Demonstrate an understanding of the workers' compensation program.
- Demonstrate an understanding of office procedures related to workers' compensation injuries/illnesses.
- Identify appropriate reporting and billing processes related to workers' compensation injuries/illnesses.
- Interpret workers' compensation forms.
- Complete a workers' compensation claim.

Exercise 1

Online Activity—Understanding Workers' Compensation

15 minutes

1. Workers' compensation is:
    a. insurance that pays medical expenses for individuals who are injured or become ill on the job.
    b. insurance that pays an individual's wages or salary if he or she becomes permanently disabled.
    c. an insurance program that protects workers from loss of income as a result of disability.
    d. a program that provides monthly cash payments to disabled individuals.

2. Workers' compensation insurance for private businesses is regulated by:
    a. county laws.
    b. state laws.
    c. federal laws.
    d. none of the above.

185

3. Federal workers' compensation laws apply to which of the following? Select all that apply.

_____ State business employees

_____ Miners

_____ Private business employees

_____ Maritime workers

_____ People who work for the government

_____ None of the above

4. Workers' compensation laws have been developed for a variety of reasons. Which of the following are purposes of workers' compensation laws? Select all that apply.

_____ To provide the best available medical care necessary, thus ensuring a prompt return to work of any injured or ill employee

_____ To provide income to the injured or ill worker—or to his or her dependents—regardless of fault

_____ To relieve public and private charities of financial drains resulting from uncompensated industrial accidents

_____ To discourage maximum employer interest in safety and rehabilitation

_____ To promote the study of causes of accidents and reduce preventable accidents and human suffering rather than concealing fault

5. Explain why workers' compensations programs are not required to comply with HIPAA standards.

6. Any abnormal condition or disorder caused by exposure to environmental factors associated with employment is referred to as an _____ illness or disease.

7. The person at the workers' compensation office who oversees the industrial case is called an _____ _____.

8. Final determination of the issues involving settlement of an industrial accident is known as _____.

9. Match the principal types of state compensation benefits to their descriptions.

**Type of State
Compensation Benefit**

_____ Medical treatment

_____ Temporary disability indemnity

_____ Permanent disability indemnity

_____ Death benefits for survivors

_____ Rehabilitation benefits

Description

a. This consists of cash payments to dependents of employees who are fatally injured.

b. This is disbursed in the form of weekly cash payments made directly to the injured or ill person.

c. This includes hospital, medical, and surgical services, medications, and prosthetic devices.

d. This can consist of medical or vocational rehabilitation in cases of severe disabilities.

e. This can consist of either weekly or monthly cash payments based on a rating system that determines the percentage of permanent disability or a lump sum award.

Exercise 2

Online Activity—Understanding Proper Office and Billing Procedures

30 minutes

- Sign in to Mountain View Clinic.
- Select **Janet Jones** from the patient list.
- Click on **Reception**.
- Under the Watch heading, click on **Patient Check-In** and watch the video.

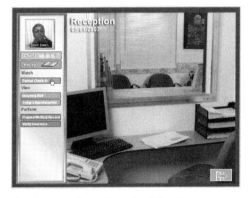

1. During check-in, what "paperwork" was Kristin referring to when she asked for documents from Ms. Jones' employer?
   a. Ms. Jones' insurance identification card.
   b. The employer's workers' compensation identification card.
   c. The patient information and problem forms.
   d. The employer's written authorization for the visit and the "Employer's Report of Occupational Injury or Illness Form."

2. Kristin did not ask Janet Jones for her insurance ID card. Was this an oversight on Kristin's part?
   a. Yes, it was an oversight.
   b. No, there is no insurance card issued for workers' compensation coverage.

3. Who is considered the responsible party in Ms. Jones' case?
   a. The patient, Janet Jones
   b. The patient's employer
   c. State health insurance
   d. Elaine Meere

4. Ms. Jones fell while stepping out of the toll booth in which she works. However, if Ms. Jones had instead fallen while going to the bank on her lunch hour to deposit money for her employer, would she have been eligible for workers' compensation benefits?
   a. No, because the accident occurred off the work site and during her lunch hour.
   b. Yes, an industrial accident does not have to occur at the customary work site. She was running a work-related errand during her lunch hour.

5. Once the physician at Mountain View Clinic is advised that Ms. Jones' injury is work-related, he must complete a:
   a. Medical Service Order.
   b. Doctor's First Report of Occupational Injury or Illness Form.
   c. Temporary Disability Form.
   d. Workers' Compensation Medical Progress Report Form.

6. The physician at Mountain View Clinic must complete all workers' compensation paperwork promptly to avoid:
   a. claim denial.
   b. any delay in income to the patient.
   c. duplicate claims submissions.
   d. penalties imposed by the Workers' Compensation Board.

7. Workers' compensation claims are forwarded by the health insurance professional to the:
   a. workers' compensation insurance carrier.
   b. workers' compensation insurance carrier and the employer.
   c. workers' compensation insurance carrier, the employer, and the state agency.
   d. workers' compensation insurance carrier, the employer, the state agency, and the patient.

8. If Janet Jones' work-related injury keeps her out of work after her initial visit to Mountain View Clinic, periodic reports must be filed to apprise the insurance carrier as to the patient's treatment plan, progress, and status. These reports are referred to as:
   a. follow-up reports.
   b. subsequent progress reports.
   c. claims for compensation.
   d. second report of injury or illness.

9. Upon Ms. Jones' return to work, the physician at Mountain View Clinic must submit a:
   a. final report.
   b. last report.
   c. summary report.
   d. final claim for compensation.

10. The charge for Janet Jones' encounter for 5/1/2007 is $160. If the workers' compensation insurer pays $135, how much can be billed to the patient?
    a. $160
    b. $25
    c. Nothing
    d. Only a copayment

11. If Ms. Jones' workers' compensation insurer does not reimburse Mountain View Clinic in a timely manner because the claim is pending, the health insurance professional:
    a. may bill the patient.
    b. may not bill the patient.

12. If Ms. Jones' workers' compensation claim is denied (as a non-work-related injury) and all efforts for appeal have been exhausted, the health insurance professional should:
    a. write off the bill.
    b. bill the patient.
    c. bill the patient or her private insurance company.

13. Because this is a work-related illness/injury, the patient will not be billed. Therefore the possibility of fraud and/or abuse is eliminated.
    a. True
    b. False

14. Ms. Jones had not previously signed a release to have bills sent to her employer and insurance company. She was not happy when she discovered that her employer would be getting a copy of this bill. If she refused to sign this release form, could Mountain View Clinic still release her information to the employer and insurance company? Explain how the receptionist should handle this situation.

15. Mountain View Clinic created a new health record (chart) and financial record (ledger) for Janet Jones' visit today. Why was this necessary?

16. In the future, Mountain View Clinic will need to be able to easily identify which of Ms. Jones' charts contains her workers' compensation record. How can this be done efficiently? Select all that apply.

_____ Front office staff will pull the charts and then decide which one is the workers' compensation chart.

_____ The medical assistant will review the charts and determine which one is the workers' compensation chart.

_____ Staff members can file the workers' compensation information in colored file folders.

_____ Colored tabs can be put on the outside of the chart to identify which is the workers' compensation chart.

➡ • Click the **X** on the video screen to close the video.
 • Click the exit arrow.
 • Click **Return to Map** and select **Yes** at the pop-up menu to return to the office map.
 • Keep **Janet Jones** as your patient and continue to the next exercise.

Exercise 3

Online Activity—Interpreting Workers' Compensation Forms

 20 minutes

• Click on **Check Out**.
• Click on **Charts**.
• Click on the **Workers' Comp** tab and select **3-First Report of Injury** or **4-Attending Physician's Report** to answer the following questions.

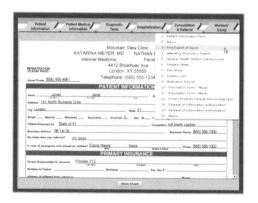

1. What is the date of Janet Jones' injury?

2. What is the OCWP file number for Janet Jones' case?

3. What is the physician's diagnosis for Janet Jones' injury?

4. What is the date of first treatment for Janet Jones' injury?

5. How did Janet Jones' injury occur?

6. Who is Janet Jones' employer?

7. What is Janet Jones' hourly wage?

8. What is Janet Jones' job title?

9. Did Janet Jones have any injury-related lost time from work?

10. Could the injury have been prevented?

11. Who is responsible for completing the Attending Physician's Report?

12. Who is responsible for completing the First Report of Injury?

→ • Leave Janet Jones' chart open and complete the next exercise.

Exercise 4

 Online Activity—Completing a Workers' Compensation Claim

 45 minutes

 1. Using the appropriate forms in Janet Jones' medical chart, along with her Encounter Form and the claims completion guidelines in Chapter 7 of your textbook, complete the claim form below.

1500

HEALTH INSURANCE CLAIM FORM

APPROVED BY NATIONAL UNIFORM CLAIM COMMITTEE 08/05

[ ] [ ] PICA

1. MEDICARE (Medicare #)	MEDICAID (Medicaid #)	TRICARE CHAMPUS (Sponsor's SSN)	CHAMPVA (Member ID#)	GROUP HEALTH PLAN (SSN or ID)	FECA BLK LUNG (SSN)	OTHER (ID)

1a. INSURED'S I.D. NUMBER (For Program in Item 1)

2. PATIENT'S NAME (Last Name, First Name, Middle Initial)

3. PATIENT'S BIRTH DATE MM DD YY   SEX M [ ] F [ ]

4. INSURED'S NAME (Last Name, First Name, Middle Initial)

5. PATIENT'S ADDRESS (No., Street)

6. PATIENT RELATIONSHIP TO INSURED   Self [ ] Spouse [ ] Child [ ] Other [ ]

7. INSURED'S ADDRESS (No., Street)

CITY   STATE

8. PATIENT STATUS   Single [ ] Married [ ] Other [ ]

CITY   STATE

ZIP CODE   TELEPHONE (Include Area Code) ( )

Employed [ ] Full-Time Student [ ] Part-Time Student [ ]

ZIP CODE   TELEPHONE (Include Area Code) ( )

9. OTHER INSURED'S NAME (Last Name, First Name, Middle Initial)

10. IS PATIENT'S CONDITION RELATED TO:

11. INSURED'S POLICY GROUP OR FECA NUMBER

a. OTHER INSURED'S POLICY OR GROUP NUMBER

a. EMPLOYMENT? (Current or Previous) YES [ ] NO [ ]

a. INSURED'S DATE OF BIRTH MM DD YY   SEX M [ ] F [ ]

b. OTHER INSURED'S DATE OF BIRTH MM DD YY   SEX M [ ] F [ ]

b. AUTO ACCIDENT?   PLACE (State)   YES [ ] NO [ ]

b. EMPLOYER'S NAME OR SCHOOL NAME

c. EMPLOYER'S NAME OR SCHOOL NAME

c. OTHER ACCIDENT? YES [ ] NO [ ]

c. INSURANCE PLAN NAME OR PROGRAM NAME

d. INSURANCE PLAN NAME OR PROGRAM NAME

10d. RESERVED FOR LOCAL USE

d. IS THERE ANOTHER HEALTH BENEFIT PLAN? YES [ ] NO [ ] *If yes*, return to and complete item 9 a-d.

READ BACK OF FORM BEFORE COMPLETING & SIGNING THIS FORM.

12. PATIENT'S OR AUTHORIZED PERSON'S SIGNATURE I authorize the release of any medical or other information necessary to process this claim. I also request payment of government benefits either to myself or to the party who accepts assignment below.

SIGNED _____   DATE _____

13. INSURED'S OR AUTHORIZED PERSON'S SIGNATURE I authorize payment of medical benefits to the undersigned physician or supplier for services described below.

SIGNED _____

14. DATE OF CURRENT MM DD YY ILLNESS (First symptom) OR INJURY (Accident) OR PREGNANCY(LMP)

15. IF PATIENT HAS HAD SAME OR SIMILAR ILLNESS GIVE FIRST DATE MM DD YY

16. DATES PATIENT UNABLE TO WORK IN CURRENT OCCUPATION MM DD YY FROM   TO MM DD YY

17. NAME OF REFERRING PROVIDER OR OTHER SOURCE

17a.

17b. NPI

18. HOSPITALIZATION DATES RELATED TO CURRENT SERVICES MM DD YY FROM   TO MM DD YY

19. RESERVED FOR LOCAL USE

20. OUTSIDE LAB? $ CHARGES   YES [ ] NO [ ]

21. DIAGNOSIS OR NATURE OF ILLNESS OR INJURY (Relate Items 1, 2, 3 or 4 to Item 24E by Line)

1. _____   3. _____

2. _____   4. _____

22. MEDICAID RESUBMISSION CODE   ORIGINAL REF. NO.

23. PRIOR AUTHORIZATION NUMBER

24. A DATE(S) OF SERVICE		B PLACE OF SERVICE	C EMG	D. PROCEDURES, SERVICES, OR SUPPLIES (Explain Unusual Circumstances)		E DIAGNOSIS POINTER	F $ CHARGES	G DAYS OR UNITS	H EPSDT Family Plan	I ID QUAL	J RENDERING PROVIDER ID #
From MM DD YY	To MM DD YY			CPT/HCPCS	MODIFIER						
1										NPI	
2										NPI	
3										NPI	
4										NPI	
5										NPI	
6										NPI	

25. FEDERAL TAX I.D. NUMBER   SSN [ ] EIN [ ]

26. PATIENT'S ACCOUNT NO.

27. ACCEPT ASSIGNMENT? (For govt. claims, see back) YES [ ] NO [ ]

28. TOTAL CHARGE $

29. AMOUNT PAID $

30. BALANCE DUE $

31. SIGNATURE OF PHYSICIAN OR SUPPLIER INCLUDING DEGREES OR CREDENTIALS (I certify that the statements on the reverse apply to this bill and are made a part thereof.)

SIGNED _____   DATE _____

32. SERVICE FACILITY LOCATION INFORMATION

33. BILLING PROVIDER INFO & PH # ( )

NUCC Instruction Manual available at: www.nucc.org   APPROVED OMB-0938-0999 FORM CMS-1500 (08/05)

• Click **Close Chart** or **Finish** to return to the Check Out area.
- Click the exit arrow.
- Click **Exit the Program** or, if continuing to a new lesson, click **Return to Map** and then click **Yes** on the pop-up menu.

Disability Income Insurance and Disability Benefit Programs

⟋◯⟍ **Reading Assignment:** Chapter 16—Disability Income Insurance and Disability Benefit Programs

Patient: Jesus Santo

Room: Reception

Objectives:

- Define the terminology associated with disability insurance.
- Identify potential disability cases.
- Identify restrictions that may prohibit a patient from receiving disability benefits.
- Understand the circumstances under which a patient would apply for either temporary or permanent disability benefits.
- Identify the claims submission process.

Exercise 1

Writing Activity—Disability Insurance Word Bank

15 minutes

Many adults with poor health are unable to work and have no income, making it difficult or even impossible to provide for themselves or their families. Often, disability insurance will replace a portion of earned income while these individuals are unable to work. It is the responsibility of the health insurance professional to assist the physician in the timely filing of disability forms and assist these patients in applying for disability benefits.

1. Match each disability-related term or abbreviation with its definition.

Definition	**Term**
_____ A program that provides monthly cash payments to low-income, elderly, blind, and/or disabled individuals	a. Armed Services Disability
	b. CSRS or FERS
_____ A program that provides monthly benefits for life to individuals who are members of the armed services on active duty who suffer a disability or illness	c. DDS
	d. Long-term disability
_____ An insurance program that protects workers from loss of income as a result of disability and provides cash benefits to disabled workers younger than 65	e. Short-term disability
	f. SSDI
_____ A team composed of a physician or psychologist and a disability examiner who will determine whether a person is eligible for Social Security disability payments	g. SSI
_____ Insurance that helps to replace income for 5 years or until the individual turns 65	
_____ The system that provides federal employees who work in civil service with disability benefits for injuries/illnesses that are not work-related	
_____ Insurance that provides an income for the early part of a disability, usually from 2 weeks to 1 year	

2. Disability insurance benefits do not provide payment for medical services to the physician. Considering this, explain why it is important for the health insurance specialist to be familiar with the terms and abbreviations defined in question 1.

Exercise 2

Online Activity—Identifying Potential Disability Cases

  20 minutes

- Sign in to Mountain View Clinic.
- Select **Jesus Santo** from the patient list.
- Click on **Reception**.
- Under the Watch heading, click on **Patient Check-In** and watch the video.

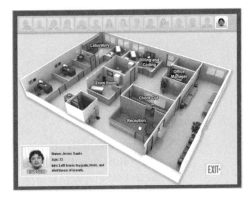

1. What is Mr. Santo's chief complaint? Does he have any additional complaints?

2. Do you see a potential disability claim on the part of Mr. Santo? What complaint could be the basis for a claim? Briefly explain your answer using some of the terms from the chapter.

3. If Mr. Santo is successful in obtaining benefits from disability income insurance, what type of benefits will he be entitled to?

4. There are several different types of disability insurance programs. Which type would best apply to Mr. Santo? Why?

5. Certain disability restrictions can affect a person's eligibility for compensation. Which of the following situations, if true, would prohibit a person from receiving disability benefits? Select all that apply.

_____ If the patient's condition is covered by workers' compensation and the rate the patient is receiving is more than the disability insurance rate

_____ If the patient's condition is covered by workers' compensation and the rate the patient is receiving is less than the disability insurance rate

_____ If the patient is receiving unemployment benefits

_____ If the patient was on strike and was injured while walking a picket line

_____ If the patient has paid into his company's voluntary disability plan and has not paid into a state fund

→ • Click the **X** on the video screen to close the video.
   • Click the exit arrow.
   • Click **Return to Map** and select **Yes** at the pop-up menu to return to the office map.
   • Keep **Jesus Santo** as your patient and continue to the next exercise.

Exercise 3

Online Activity—Temporary Versus Permanent Disability

15 minutes

- Click on **Check Out**.
- Click on **Charts**.
- Click on the **Patient Medical Information** tab and select **1-Progress Notes**.
- Read the notes from 5/1/06.

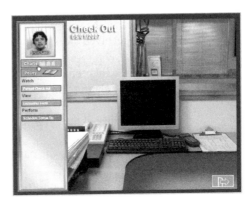

1. Temporary disability exists when a person cannot perform all the functions of his or her

   regular job for a _____ period of time.

2. The definition for total disability _____ from policy to policy.

3. Dr. Meyers has listed several diagnoses in Mr. Santo's chart that have the potential to become very serious and possibly disabling if left untreated. Identify these diagnoses in the list below. Select all that apply.

   _____ Shortness of breath

   _____ Fatigue

   _____ Cellulitis

   _____ Reactive airway disease

   _____ COPD

   _____ Diarrhea

   _____ Vomiting

4. Let's assume that Mr. Santo's condition becomes worse and he must be admitted to the hospital for IV antibiotics. If he is hospitalized for 14 days and out of work for 30 full days, which of the following would best describe his case?
   a. Temporary, because he is currently able to return to work
   b. Permanent, because he may be out of work in the future for the same condition
   c. Permanent, because he was out of work for 30 full days

- Click **Close Chart** to return to the Check Out area.
- Click the exit arrow.
- Click **Exit the Program** or, if continuing to a new lesson, click **Return to Map** and then click **Yes** on the pop-up menu.

Exercise 4

 Online Activity—The Claims Submission Process

 10 minutes

1. Which of the following steps should you, as the insurance billing specialist, take after you have received a disability income claim form for Mr. Santo? Select all that apply.

    _____ Be prepared to extract data from source documents to assist in completion of the claim form

    _____ Read the information carefully and sign the document on behalf of the physician

    _____ Interview the patient's employer for wage statements

    _____ Review the form to ensure that all required areas have been completed by the physician

    _____ Assist in submitting the form within the appropriate time limits

    _____ Confirm that the patient has signed an authorization form to release medical information

Hospital Billing

 Reading Assignment: Chapter 17—Hospital Billing

Patient: Wilson Metcalf

Rooms: Reception, Exam Room, Check Out

Objectives:

- Define appropriateness evaluation protocols and understand how they are used to screen for admission.
- Explain the admitting procedure for a Medicare patient to ensure that insurance guidelines are met.
- Understand the inpatient billing process.

Exercise 1

 Online Activity—Appropriateness Evaluation Protocols

15 minutes

- Sign in to Mountain View Clinic.
- Select **Wilson Metcalf** from the patient list.
- Click on **Reception**.
- Under the Watch heading, click on **Patient Check-In** and watch the video.

1. Dr. Meyer decides that he must admit Mr. Metcalf. However, the admission must first meet the hospital's Appropriateness Evaluation Protocols (AEPs). What does this mean?
   a. Dr. Meyer must evaluate Mr. Metcalf to determine whether or not the hospital will allow him to be admitted.
   b. Dr. Meyer must be certified to admit patients into the hospital appropriately.
   c. The hospital must meet certain standards certifying that Mr. Metcalf's complaints warrant admission to the hospital.
   d. Mr. Metcalf must sign a certification stating that he has insurance that will provide appropriate insurance coverage during his hospital stay.

2. Mr. Metcalf has Medicare insurance, which requires that all patients meet at least one severity of illness or intensity of service criterion to be certified for admission and reimbursement. Using the AEP chart in the textbook, what sign or symptom does Mr. Metcalf have that will support his admission?
   a. Sudden onset of unconsciousness or disorientation
   b. Pulse rate <50 or >140
   c. Sudden onset of loss of sight
   d. Active, uncontrolled bleeding

3. Who will review the documentation in Mr. Metcalf's medical record within the first 24 hours, to ensure that the admission was appropriate?
   a. Dr. Meyer
   b. The health insurance professional
   c. American Hospital Association
   d. The hospital's utilization review department

* Click the **X** on the video screen to close the video.
* Click the exit arrow.
* Click **Return to Map** and select **Yes** at the pop-up menu to return to the office map.
* Keep **Wilson Metcalf** as your patient and continue to the next exercise.

Exercise 2

Online Activity—Admitting Procedures for Medicare and Major Insurance Programs

 40 minutes

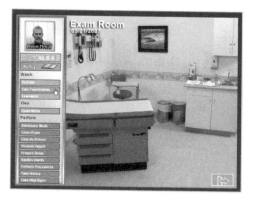

* Click on **Exam Room**.
* Under the Watch heading, click on **Care Coordination** and watch the video.
* Click the **X** on the video screen to close the video.
* Under the Watch heading, click on **Teamwork** and watch the video.
* Click the **X** on the video screen to close the video.
* Click the exit arrow.
* Click **Return to Map** and select **Yes** at the pop-up menu to return to the office map.
* Keep **Wilson Metcalf** as your patient
* Click on **Check Out** on the office map.
* Under the Watch heading, click on **Patient Check-Out** and watch the video.
* Click the **X** on the video screen to close the video.

- Click on the **Encounter Form** clipboard and review.
- Click **Finish** to return to the Check Out area.
- Click on **Charts**.
- Click on the **Patient Medical Information** tab, and select **1-Progress Notes**.

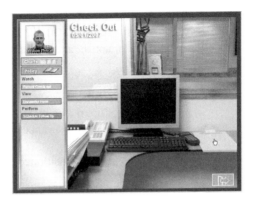

1. Which diagnoses documented in Mr. Metcalf's Progress Notes will most likely be used as the admitting diagnoses when he arrives at the hospital? Select all that apply.

   _____ Alcoholic hepatitis/cirrhosis

   _____ Calf tenderness

   _____ Hemorrhoids

   _____ Jaundiced sclera

   _____ Muscle wasting

   _____ Prostate enlargement

   _____ Pruritus

   _____ R/O liver abscess

   _____ Severe hydration and malnutrition

   _____ Testicular varicoceles

2. The definition of *principal diagnosis* is:
   a. the principal reason that the patient sought care.
   b. the condition established after study that is chiefly responsible for admission to the hospital.
   c. the signs and symptoms present on admission.
   d. all conditions that will be ruled out during the patient's hospital stay.

3. A _____ _____ _____ will be used to verify Mr. Metcalf's Medicare coverage.

4. The hospital where Mr. Metcalf is admitted must comply with Medicare. One of these rules states that if Mr. Metcalf receives diagnostic tests or any other hospital services within

   _____ hours of his admission to the hospital, then all such services will be

   _____ with the inpatient services as long as they are related to his admission.

5. If the Medicare rule in the previous question is not complied with, it may be considered

fraud or abuse, and violation would result in a penalty of _____ or

_____.

6. Which of the major insurance programs require admitting personnel to obtain a photocopy of the patient's insurance card (front and back)? Select all that apply.

_____ Private insurance

_____ Managed care organizations

_____ Medicaid

_____ Medicare

_____ TRICARE and CHAMPVA

_____ Workers' compensation

7. Which of the major insurance programs require admitting personnel to obtain prior authorization? Select all that apply.

_____ Private insurance

_____ Managed care organizations

_____ Medicaid

_____ Medicare

_____ TRICARE and CHAMPVA

_____ Workers' compensation

8. If Mr. Metcalf has a catheter-associated urinary tract infection at the time he is admitted,

it should be reported with a _____ indicator code, because Medicare will not pay for it if it is acquired during his hospital inpatient stay.

→ • Click **Close Chart** to return to the Check Out area.
 • Click the exit arrow.
 • Click **Exit the Program** or, if continuing to a new lesson, click **Return to Map** and then click **Yes** on the pop-up menu.

Exercise 3

Writing Activity—Understanding the Inpatient Billing Process

30 minutes

1. Identify the roles and responsibilities of the various hospital staff and/or departments involved in the process of billing for Mr. Metcalf's inpatient stay.

Role/Responsibilities	Hospital Staff and/or Department
_____ Will verify the physician's orders and the medical record against each charge item on Mr. Metcalf's bill	a. Admitting clerk
	b. Insurance verifier
_____ Will read Mr. Metcalf's photocopied insurance ID card and call the physician for additional information, if needed	c. Attending physician
	d. Transcriptionist
_____ Will check the completeness of Mr. Metcalf's medical record for dictated reports and signatures	e. Discharge analyst
	f. CDM committee
_____ Will dictate the history and physical performed on Mr. Metcalf on admission	g. Code specialist
_____ Will interview Mr. Metcalf to obtain the personal and insurance information needed to bill for services performed	h. Insurance billing editor
	i. Nurse auditor
_____ Will assist physicians in preparing written medical records for services received while Mr. Metcalf is an inpatient	
_____ Will be responsible for keeping the coding database (which is used to report Mr. Metcalf's services) current and accurate	
_____ Will review the hospital's electronic claim form to ensure it is complete and accurate	
_____ Will abstract procedures and diagnoses from Mr. Metcalf's medical record and assign the appropriate codes for services provided	

2. The institutional uniform claim form developed by the National Uniform Billing Committee that will be used to report Mr. Metcalf's inpatient stay is referred to as the _____.

3. The claim form used to report hospital and other institutional services has _____ form locators (fields).

4. The field on the claim form that is to report the hospital's federal tax ID number is

_____.

5. The field on the hospital's claim form that is used to report the time Mr. Metcalf was admitted to the hospital for inpatient care is _____.

6. The field on the hospital's claim form that is used to report the time Mr. Metcalf was discharged from the hospital is _____.

7. The field on the hospital's claim form that is used to report the principal diagnosis code for Mr. Metcalf is _____.

8. The field on the hospital's claim form that is used to report the admitting diagnosis for Mr. Metcalf is _____.

9. The field on the hospital's claim form that is used to report the codes for the principal procedures performed on Mr. Metcalf is _____.

10. Diagnosis coding sequence is important in the billing of Mr. Metcalf's hospital inpatient stay because maximum payment is based on the _____ system, which bases payment on fixed dollar amounts for the principal diagnosis listed.

11. Which of the following situations, if they occurred, would be likely to result in allegations of fraud and abuse? Select all that apply.

    _____ Mr. Metcalf receives a hospital bill that has items listed on it with no explanation or description of what the charges are for.

    _____ Mr. Metcalf contacts the hospital billing department because his statement has no explanations of charges, and he is told that the hospital will have to charge him a fee for a more detailed statement.

    _____ Mr. Metcalf notices that he is being billed for a blood transfusion that he did not receive.

    _____ Mr. Metcalf's son reviews the Medicare EOB and notices that his father was charged for a colonoscopy that he refused to have.

LESSON 18

Seeking a Job and Attaining Professional Advancement

 Reading Assignment: Chapter 18—Seeking a Job and
Attaining Professional Advancement

Patients: John R. Simmons, Rhea Davison

Rooms: Reception, Check Out

Objectives:

- Prepare to conduct a job search.
- Understand the interview process.
- Identify the level of professionalism required during the interview process.
- Create a professional resume, cover letter, and follow-up letter.
- Understand the types of certifications available to individuals for professional advancement.

 Exercise 1

Writing Activity—Preparing to Conduct a Job Search

15 minutes

1. Listed below are several methods of conducting a job search. From this list, select the three methods that you think you would prefer to use for a job search. Be prepared to explain your choices during class discussion.
   a. Contact your school's placement personnel
   b. Join a professional organization to network with others
   c. Attend a community job fair
   d. Review the local newspaper
   e. Conduct an online job search
   f. Contact or talk with people currently employed at an office, hospital, insurance company, or association
   g. Make unannounced visits ("cold calls") to job locations
   h. Visit or contact the local medical society's office
   i. Send "blind" mailings to potential employers
   j. Search for part-time employment that might lead to a permanent full-time position

207

2. Indicate whether each of the following statements regarding completion of an application form is true or false.

   a. _____ When completing an application, your ability to follow directions is extremely important.

   b. _____ It is typically recommended that applications be completed in pencil so that any error can be erased easily and corrected.

   c. _____ Dates of employment at previous jobs do not have to be exact or completely accurate, because employers do not typically confirm them.

   d. _____ When a question is asked about salary requirements, it is acceptable to answer "Negotiable."

   e. _____ Accuracy and legible handwriting are extremely important.

   f. _____ A previously prepared resume can be helpful to use a reference while completing applications.

   g. _____ It is not acceptable to write "NA" (not applicable) if a question does not apply to your situation.

3. Below, identify the correct description for each of the elements needed to prepare for your job search.

Description	Element Required for the Job Search
_____ The data sheet designed to "sell" your job qualifications to a prospective employer	a. Interview
_____ An explanation of how your qualifications and skills will benefit the prospective employer	b. Portfolio
_____ An organized file of your letters of recommendations, names of references, and copies of certifications	c. Cover letter
_____ A formal consultation during which a prospective employer asks you questions to evaluate your qualifications	d. Follow-up letter
_____ An opportunity to restate your interest in a position and to keep your name before the potential employer	e. Resume

Exercise 2

Online Activity—Understanding the Interview Process

 20 minutes

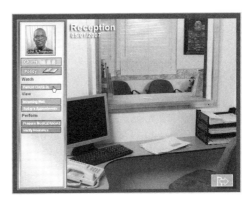

- Sign in to Mountain View Clinic.
- Select **John R. Simmons** from the patient list.
- Click on **Reception**.
- Under the Watch heading, click on **Patient Check-In** and watch the video. Pay close attention to the conversation between Katie and Dr. Simmons once he sits down.

1. It is a well-known fact that an applicant makes either a positive or negative impression in the first 30 seconds after walking through the door for an interview. Do you think Katie made a good first impression with the receptionist and/or office manager? Why or why not?

2. What were some of the unprofessional things Katie said to Dr. Simmons in the waiting room?

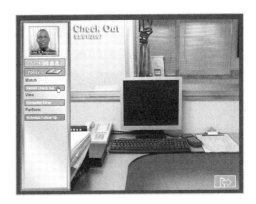

- Click the **X** on the video screen to close the video.
- Click the exit arrow.
- Click **Return to Map** and select **Yes** at the pop-up menu to return to the office map.
- Click on **Check Out**.
- Under the Watch heading, click on **Patient Check-Out** and watch the video.

3. Dr. Simmons asks the receptionist whether he will be seeing the same medical assistant on his next visit or whether he can ask for a different one. What was his concern?

4. Assume that you are the office manager and you have heard the conversation between Katie and Dr. Simmons in the waiting room, as well as Dr. Simmons' concerns at check-out. Would you be inclined to hire Katie? Explain your answer.

5. Indicate whether each of the following statements regarding the interview process is true or false.

   a. _____ When multiple applicants have similar skills and education, the decision to hire is frequently based on physical appearance at the interview.

   b. _____ It is important to show an intense interest in the benefits that are offered by the prospective employer.

   c. _____ Research has shown that a good time to schedule an interview is 4:00 p.m. on a Friday.

   d. _____ A suggested method to prepare for an interview is role-playing.

   e. _____ Questions regarding your personal life and provisions for child care are acceptable and must be answered during an interview.

   f. _____ If you are asked questions regarding age, ethnic background, or physical problems, it is acceptable to answer, "I think that question is irrelevant to the requirements of this position."

   g. _____ Shaking hands at the end of the interview is not recommended, because it may seem overly assertive.

→ • Click the **X** on the video screen to close the video.
   • Click the exit arrow.
   • Click **Return to Map** and select **Yes** at the pop-up menu to return to the office map.

Exercise 3

 Writing Activity—Creating a Professional Resume, Cover Letter, and Follow-Up Letter

 45 minutes

 Mountain View Clinic has a job opening. Read the advertisement and job description below to answer the questions in this exercise. Refer to your textbook for help, if needed.

> Position Available: Insurance Billing Specialist. Full-time position.
>
> Job duties will include the following: Files all insurance claims to contracted insurance carriers. Tracks the status of all claims and resubmits as appropriate. Mails monthly patient statements. Assigns all ICD-9-CM and CPT codes to Encounter Forms, checking against documentation. Responsible for follow-up on overdue accounts for collection.
>
> Applicant should possess excellent communication and problem-solving skills, computer experience, and knowledge of ICD-9-CM and CPT coding. Two years of experience in a physician's office preferred.
>
> Please send your resume, salary requirements, and references to Mountain View Clinic, Attn: Elizabeth Brown, Office Manager, PO Box 2551, London, XY 55555.

1. You have decided to apply for the opening! First, you need to prepare your resume. Using the information in the job advertisement, prepare a draft of your resume below.

2. You know that a cover letter (letter of introduction) is important to get the employer to take notice of your application. Using the information provided in the job advertisement for Mountain View Clinic, prepare a draft of your cover letter below.

3. Your interview went well, but you want to make the best impression by sending a follow-up letter. Using the contact information provided in the Mountain View Clinic advertisement, prepare a draft of your follow-up letter below.

Exercise 4

 Online Activity—Understanding the Types of Certification Available for Professional Advancement

 20 minutes

- Select **Rhea Davison** from the patient list.
- Click on **Reception**.
- Under the Watch heading, click on **Patient Check-In** and watch the video.
- **Stop** the video once Kristen finishes her conversation regarding certification.

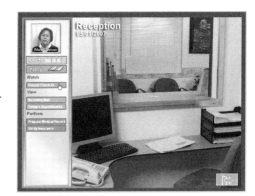

1. Kristin tells Ms. Davison that she is "certified." What does it mean to be "certified"?

2. Once certified, you are a member of a professional organization. What are some advantages of membership? Select all that apply.

_____ Helps to keep you up to date on information regarding your field

_____ Provides continuing education

_____ Provides a link for further employment opportunities

_____ Makes you look good to other staff members

_____ Allows you to receive newsletters and journals for further education

_____ Allows you to attend local meetings with guest speakers on topics of current interest

For questions 3, 4, and 5 below, refer to the listing of certifications and registrations provided in your textbook.

3. Explain the difference between CPC and CPC-H.

4. Explain the difference between the CCS and CCS-P.

5. Identify which credential(s) you would be interested in obtaining to advance your career further. Explain your reasons.

- Click the **X** on the video screen to close the video.
- Click the exit arrow.
- Click **Exit the Program**.

1500

HEALTH INSURANCE CLAIM FORM

APPROVED BY NATIONAL UNIFORM CLAIM COMMITTEE 08/05

□□□ PICA			PICA □□□

CARRIER

1. MEDICARE MEDICAID TRICARE CHAMPUS CHAMPVA GROUP HEALTH PLAN FECA BLK LUNG OTHER	1a. INSURED'S I.D. NUMBER (For Program in Item 1)
□ (Medicare #) □ (Medicaid #) □ (Sponsor's SSN) □ (Member ID#) □ (SSN or ID) □ (SSN) □ (ID)	

2. PATIENT'S NAME (Last Name, First Name, Middle Initial)	3. PATIENT'S BIRTH DATE MM DD YY SEX M □ F □	4. INSURED'S NAME (Last Name, First Name, Middle Initial)

5. PATIENT'S ADDRESS (No., Street)	6. PATIENT RELATIONSHIP TO INSURED Self □ Spouse □ Child □ Other □	7. INSURED'S ADDRESS (No., Street)

CITY	STATE	8. PATIENT STATUS Single □ Married □ Other □	CITY	STATE

ZIP CODE	TELEPHONE (Include Area Code) ( )	Employed □ Full-Time Student □ Part-Time Student □	ZIP CODE	TELEPHONE (Include Area Code) ( )

9. OTHER INSURED'S NAME (Last Name, First Name, Middle Initial)	10. IS PATIENT'S CONDITION RELATED TO:	11. INSURED'S POLICY GROUP OR FECA NUMBER

a. OTHER INSURED'S POLICY OR GROUP NUMBER	a. EMPLOYMENT? (Current or Previous) □ YES □ NO	a. INSURED'S DATE OF BIRTH MM DD YY SEX M □ F □

b. OTHER INSURED'S DATE OF BIRTH MM DD YY SEX M □ F □	b. AUTO ACCIDENT? □ YES □ NO PLACE (State)	b. EMPLOYER'S NAME OR SCHOOL NAME

c. EMPLOYER'S NAME OR SCHOOL NAME	c. OTHER ACCIDENT? □ YES □ NO	c. INSURANCE PLAN NAME OR PROGRAM NAME

d. INSURANCE PLAN NAME OR PROGRAM NAME	10d. RESERVED FOR LOCAL USE	d. IS THERE ANOTHER HEALTH BENEFIT PLAN? □ YES □ NO If yes, return to and complete item 9 a-d.

READ BACK OF FORM BEFORE COMPLETING & SIGNING THIS FORM.

12. PATIENT'S OR AUTHORIZED PERSON'S SIGNATURE I authorize the release of any medical or other information necessary to process this claim. I also request payment of government benefits either to myself or to the party who accepts assignment below.	13. INSURED'S OR AUTHORIZED PERSON'S SIGNATURE I authorize payment of medical benefits to the undersigned physician or supplier for services described below.
SIGNED_____ DATE_____	SIGNED_____

PATIENT AND INSURED INFORMATION

14. DATE OF CURRENT MM DD YY ILLNESS (First symptom) OR INJURY (Accident) OR PREGNANCY(LMP)	15. IF PATIENT HAS HAD SAME OR SIMILAR ILLNESS GIVE FIRST DATE MM DD YY	16. DATES PATIENT UNABLE TO WORK IN CURRENT OCCUPATION MM DD YY MM DD YY FROM TO

17. NAME OF REFERRING PROVIDER OR OTHER SOURCE	17a.	18. HOSPITALIZATION DATES RELATED TO CURRENT SERVICES MM DD YY MM DD YY FROM TO
	17b. NPI	

19. RESERVED FOR LOCAL USE	20. OUTSIDE LAB? □ YES □ NO $ CHARGES

21. DIAGNOSIS OR NATURE OF ILLNESS OR INJURY (Relate Items 1, 2, 3 or 4 to Item 24E by Line)	22. MEDICAID RESUBMISSION CODE ORIGINAL REF. NO.
1. _____ 3. _____	
2. _____ 4. _____	23. PRIOR AUTHORIZATION NUMBER

24. A. DATE(S) OF SERVICE From To MM DD YY MM DD YY	B. PLACE OF SERVICE	C. EMG	D. PROCEDURES, SERVICES, OR SUPPLIES (Explain Unusual Circumstances) CPT/HCPCS MODIFIER	E. DIAGNOSIS POINTER	F. $ CHARGES	G. DAYS OR UNITS	H. EPSDT Family Plan	I. ID QUAL	J. RENDERING PROVIDER ID. #
1								NPI	
2								NPI	
3								NPI	
4								NPI	
5								NPI	
6								NPI	

25. FEDERAL TAX I.D. NUMBER SSN EIN □ □	26. PATIENT'S ACCOUNT NO.	27. ACCEPT ASSIGNMENT? (For govt. claims, see back) □ YES □ NO	28. TOTAL CHARGE $	29. AMOUNT PAID $	30. BALANCE DUE $

31. SIGNATURE OF PHYSICIAN OR SUPPLIER INCLUDING DEGREES OR CREDENTIALS (I certify that the statements on the reverse apply to this bill and are made a part thereof.) SIGNED_____ DATE_____	32. SERVICE FACILITY LOCATION INFORMATION a. b.	33. BILLING PROVIDER INFO & PH # ( ) a. b.

PHYSICIAN OR SUPPLIER INFORMATION

NUCC Instruction Manual available at: www.nucc.org   APPROVED OMB-0938-0999 FORM CMS-1500 (08/05)

Mountain View Clinic
Patient Ledger

DATE:

Patient ID:

Patient Name:

Insurance Type:

Date	Professional Service	Fee ($)	Payment ($)	Adj. ($)	Prev. Bal. ($)	New Balance ($)
Totals						

Mountain View Clinic
Daysheet

Date	Professional Service	Fee	Payment	Adjustment	New Balance	Old Balance	Patient's Name	Distribution	
								Dr. Hayler	Dr. Meyer
TOTALS								**TOTALS**	

PRIMARY INSURANCE

Person Responsible for Account _____ _____ _____
                                                   Last Name   First Name   Initial

Relation to Patient _____ Birthdate _____ Soc. Sec.#

Address (if different from patient's) _____ Phone _____

City _____ State _____ Zip _____

Person Responsible Employed by _____ Occupation _____

Business Address _____ Business Phone _____

Insurance Company _____

Contract # _____ Group # _____ Subscriber # _____

Name of other dependents covered under this plan _____

ADDITIONAL INSURANCE

Is patient covered by additional insurance? _____ Yes _____ No

Subscriber Name _____ Birthdate _____ Relation to Patient _____

Address (if different from patient's) _____ Phone _____

City _____ State _____ Zip _____

Subscriber Employed by _____ Business Phone _____

Insurance Company _____ Soc. Sec.# _____

Contract # _____ Group # _____ Subscriber # _____

Name of other dependents covered under this plan _____